The Journey Continues

Alzheimer's Trippin'
with George

*Over The Bumps
With Friends, Family and Community Support*

By SUSAN STRALEY

Copyright © 2019 by Susan Straley

All rights reserved. No part of this book may be reproduced in any form or by any electronic or mechanical means, including information storage and retrieval systems, without permission in writing from the author, except by reviewers, who may quote brief passages in a review.

ISBN-13: 978-1-7335465-3-9

Cover design by Landofawes
Photo front cover by Larry Varney
Edited by Margaret Juhl and Mary McNeece

Printed in United States of America

Independently Published
Ingramspark and Amazon

Susan@susanstraley.com

www.susanstraley.com

Dedication

Dedicated to:

Dementia Divas and Dancing Goddesses everywhere
and to Caregiving Princes;

All of you who have in the past and will in the future reach out to
help someone who is caregiving;

My awesome sister, Mary McCarren, and
The Withlacoochee Bicycle Riders – you make life fun!

Acknowledgments

This story might have been a sad one if it weren't for the love and support of so many in our life. Instead, it turned into a love story – a story of people coming together to lift us up and carry us through. Thanks to our friends and family who helped in many, many ways. Thanks for the meals, the hugs, the words of encouragement, the invitations, the shelter, the fun, the laughter, the lifting, the repairs, the labor and the donations.

I am afraid to name you all. I fear I will forget one who did so much. There are so many to thank!

A special thanks to Debra and Glen Alford for making this "trip" so much more fun than it would have been without your: scrumptious meals; trips; good-times; understanding; laughter; companionship; my purple trike; and a bed when I needed one.

Thanks to those who fed us and housed us on our trips, supported us with hugs, kept us in their lives socially, helped with our move to our new home, did handyman work, provided respite care, sent cards, gave gifts, and made calls.

Thanks to: my awesome sister, Mary, and her husband Dave; friends Mark and Jane Blackman; Sandy and John Schultz; Kathi Sieger; Jodie and Carl Ralston; Frankie and Dennis Newcom; Louise and Richard Patenaude; Margaret and Zip Juhl; Jennifer and David Aggett; Regis and Cindy Hampton; Ralph and Kathy Burns; Dick Marr; Mari Towle; Jerry Willert; Wilma and Hesh Ackerman; Ann and Fred Abeles; Kay and Jim Dunn; Audrey Bunchkowski; Connie and Jerry Tice; Diane Jacobson; Maryann Radscheid; Ken and Judy Parker; Preston Watters; Becky Martin; Dennis Reiland; Jane Simmons; Charlotte Key; Norma Scott; Colleen and Tony Balock; Connie Rubis; Jeremy and Mel Dickinson; Beth and Jim Richardson; Nancy and Don Purcell; Barbara Cabrera; Doyle Rabjon; Beverly Lynde.

Thanks to the generosity of all those who pitched in to keep us riding, especially: Bill and Christine Delouche; Cindy and Regis Hampton; Rolf and Barbara Garthus; Gene and Linda Craig; Richard Patenaude; Zip Juhl; the staff at Trailside Bike; and so many more who donated toward the tandem project.

I would have been lost without the people in the community that provided education, advice, and direction. Thanks to: Debbie

Selsavage; Theressa Foster; Karen Kline and her team of wonderful volunteers at Memory Lane; and all of the Dementia Divas and Amazing Princes.

A special thanks to Divas, Dianne Terry and Karon Wolfe. They provided support and encouragement to move forward in turning the journal into a book.

There are so many more, those who used my transport services and house watching and pet watching services so I could make a few dollars while being there for George.

Thanks to Mary and Margaret, my friendly editors who read carefully through both <u>Alzheimer's Trippin'</u> books to check my spelling and grammar. Any errors you, the reader, have found were because I kept making changes after they were done. Sorry!

Thank you to all of you readers. Thanks for "Trippin'" with us.

Table of Contents`

Background..1
The Alzheimer's Roller Coaster 3
Goofin' up – Fixin' up 4
Money Money 12
Hurricane Matthew....................................17
Downsizing...19
Fun While Living With Alzheimer's 24
Trying to Maintain the Status Quo 31
   Ladies Night..31
   Traveling..32
Dementia Caregivers Stuff Feelings 36
The Art of Dealing with Bullies...............45
   The Bully Encounter..........................45
   Pooh Goo 46
   Day Care 47
   Airbnb...47
   Friends Help 48
   In-home Help Is Coming...................49
It's Good, It's Bad, It Just Is 51
   Education..53
   Blessed With Good Friends..............54
   Counting Blessings............................56
Lucky Enough To Be SAVVY 59
   SAVVY Caregiver Training..............61
   Levels and Stages of Dementia.........62
   What Else?...63
Towels and Pre-arrangements 67

> Towels 67
> Pre-arrangements 69
> Keeping Active 70
> In Home Respite Care 73
> Shadowing 74

Feels Like a Speeding Train 75

> Symptoms of Decline 76
> Respite Care Adjustments 77
> Getting Organized 78

Enjoying Our Moments 80

> Respite Care Rescue 82
> Traveling With Dementia 83
> Margarita Surprise 83

We Are The Fortunate Ones! 84

> Flight to Wisconsin 84
> Scent Kit 87
> Preparing the Heart and Mind 88

Life in Snippets 90

> "I Have Dementia" 90
> Preparing for What's Ahead 91
> Words Are Lost 93
> Bus and Help 93
> Sometimes Capacities Are Unknown 93
> Life Still Interrupts 94

"Will You PLEASE Just Sit and Stay Already?" 95

> Caregiver Pointers 96

Riding the waves of Dementia and Caregiving 100
Dementia Care Training and Still Saying Goodbye. 103

> Caregiver Training 105
> Caregiving Pointers 106
> Work 109
> It's All About ME! 110

Alzheimer's Care Sparks Escape From Hurricane...111
Evacuation Fun..113
Travel Challenges..117
Roaming Rome...122
Head for the Hills!...125
Sub-surface Scream of Frustration............................127
A Brighter Day After the Whine................................131
Surprise! We are heading your way..........................135
Joy of Traveling with George....................................138
Beautiful Fall Day...144
Great Days Full Of "No!" "Don't..." "Stop!"..........146
Fortunate Encounters..151
Sleep Deprived Caregiver Grumbles........................154
A Peek into George's Sorrow....................................158
Up Over the Lake -- Mackinaw City........................162
Mackinac Island..166
Bicycle Friends are the Best!....................................169
Trike Ride in Indiana..172
South...175
Zoo Stop and a Mishap...179
Back Home..183
Caregiver: Entertainment Engineer, Snot Cop........188
   Respite..190
   Going Bonkers..192
   More Happenings...194
   Snot Cop...199
   Poop Police..199
Dementia DooDoo Diva...201
   Alzheimer's is Crappy..201
   Respect..201
   Things That I Have Tried....................................203
   Transition to Diapers..203
   Checking For Pooh..204
   Incontinence Supplies...205
   To Go Bags..208

- Step by Step..208
- Instructing Respite Caregivers 210

More of Living -- Good Ol' Days.............................211
- Alzheimer's Disease Kills 211
- Memory Care Decisions..212
- Seeking Income Production....................................212
- Life is good!..213
- In The News 221

AAAAAAAhhhhhhhhhhh 223
- VA Provides Supplies!!!......................................224
- Changes..227

Sleep, the Game Changer 228
Love Beneath Us..230
- I Get Away!..230
- Tandem Love..232

Our First E-assist Tandem Rides 235
- Group Ride Number One..237

Back In The Saddle..240
- Support Group 242
- Dealing With Death 243
- Symptoms Increase..243
- George's Memorial Trike......................................244
- Naming the Trike...244

Applause and Tears..246
- Sister Visit...247
- Disease Is Nibbling Away.....................................250

A Not So Typical Morning....................................251
- Still Having Fun...255

Through Decline, Glimpses of George 256
Falling Forward 261

Witness To A Fall 261
Spiffing Up My Old Trike 262
Renter Update, Warm Showers 264
   Renter Update 264
   Alzheimer's Symptoms 265
   Trike painted 267
   This week 268
My Sweet George, Gone Too Soon 270
Friends, Family, Therapy and Sleep-overs 273
The Essence of George 277
Resources 286
About the Author 288

Background

"Surround yourself with love."
Dove candy wrapper

George grew a career as an engineer and a Wisconsin business owner. He was well-respected among his peers during his career. He loved computer programming and mechanical engineering.

In 2008 he lost interest in working his business and we semi-retired to Florida. We chose Inverness, a small town on the Withlacoochee bike trail, a 46-mile trail shaded by huge oak trees with swaying Spanish moss. Right away we started riding with a group of bikers called the Withlacoochee Bicycle Riders (WBR). We didn't know then how much this group of people would be part of the village it takes to care for someone with dementia.

In 2011 George let me take over as owner and president of the company he had built, something that seemed strange to me at the time, but I thought he was just "burned out" and ready to retire.

It wasn't until 2014 that I saw symptoms of dementia so blatant that I could not deny what was happening.

After many tests to find the cause and eliminate other causes, George was finally definitively diagnosed in June of 2015 with neutral pressure hydrocephalus and possibly Alzheimer's disease. With hydrocephalus, doctors may try putting a stent into the brain to drain the fluid if they think it will help with the cognitive ability. After testing they concluded it would not help George.

The prognosis is that brain cells die, cognitive abilities diminish. Death comes sometimes within a few years; sometimes the disease can take over 20 years to claim its victim.

In an effort to live our remaining time together as fully as possible, I drove us around parts of the United States in 2016, visiting friends and family and sites. I kept a blog/journal to keep my friends and family informed of how we were doing. The journal became a way to share the joy of our discoveries as well as communicate the experiences of loving and caring for someone with dementia.

When we returned home from our trip, readers of the blog encouraged me to keep writing and sharing. They didn't want the journey to end, and in reality, our discoveries and new experiences continued. I found the journal/blog was a way for me to reach out, maintain sanity, and share the blessings of the long slow goodbye to George.

It is not necessary to read the first book in the Trippin' Series to understand, enjoy, and learn from this book. But if you would like to experience our trip with us, I encourage you to read *Alzheimer's Trippin' with George: Diagnosis to Discovery in 10,000 Miles.* You will find many joy-filled moments interspersed with caregiving tips.

This book that you hold in your hands begins where the previous book left off. Our story and your adventure with us, it didn't end… *The Journey Continues.*

The Alzheimer's Roller Coaster

Sunday, September 4, 2016

The cruelest part of dementia for loved ones, I think, is the roller coaster. Just when you are feeling adjusted to the loss of your loved one, they have a great day.

George is back! He speaks with a strong voice; he laughs his full, joyful laugh. I fall in love all over again.

Then, I get to experience loss again when he fades once more into the misty, foggy world of the demented brain.

Other caregivers tell stories of their loved ones getting mean and violent, and two minutes later they are their sweet selves. The family members' hearts are racing, and they are fighting back fear, sorrow, even hate; yet they can't express any of it because the person with the dementia has forgotten all about their outburst.

How does that happen? If the brain cells are dead like the doctors say, then how can someone who couldn't carry on a conversation for many weeks now all of a sudden be able to chat with you? Someone who can't think what to do with themselves now thinks to take out the trash and the recycling.

We are back from traveling for three months. Over that time I have witnessed little losses in George's abilities.

Our journey doesn't end. It continues but with less driving.

He had good days when we were traveling. So this peek at who he was is not due to the familiar surroundings.

I have heard of people on their deathbeds. Then just before they die they have a day where they sit up in bed and have conversations and seem so much better.

The brain is one strange organ. It is a mystery.

Goofin' Up – Fixin' Up

We arrived home last week from our long trip.

Upon sifting through the junk mail that was not forwarded to us on the trip, I found a few surprises. A big one was the joint account, our main checking account that had automatic bill-paying set up, was closed because I had turned in POA papers to the bank that were not correctly filled out.

Another surprise was a notice in the mail that George's health insurance was canceled because I didn't pay the premium. The premium wasn't paid because our bank had closed the account.

On Thursday morning, as soon as the clock said the bank was open, I called. I talked to someone and told them our story, and they said they could not make the account they had shut off active again. So I pushed and prodded, but then I finally asked, "Well, what do I do now?" and just then our connection ended.

I screamed at the phone.

"AAAAAAAAAAAAHHHHHHHH," I yelled. "HOW CAN I FIX THIS??? AAAAAAAAAA." Then I saw George standing by me watching, and I looked at him and smiled and started laughing at myself.

I stood up and hugged him and laughed; then the laughs turned into sobs. I was crying! Not a little weep but a huge dribbly honking loud release. George started crying too... but he was quiet about it.

I went and blew my nose. I was shocked. I thought I was handling things pretty well. Where did *that* come from???

As much as we didn't want to get in the car right away again, I had to drive to the bank and the insurance office to get things straightened out.

Fortunately, there is a Blue Cross office in Inverness. The agent told me not to worry. He said there is a grace period. He let me call from his office phone to pay the bills that were behind and keep George's insurance. It was a relief to have that taken care of.

Our bank is in Ocala... The Villages, actually. I thought I was driving the right way up 41 and 200. But when I started entering Ocala I realized I had gone the wrong way. We were supposed to take 44 East!

I pulled out the iPad. We were 45 minutes away from the bank, probably further away than from our home. Sigh. More driving....

At the bank we opened another account with George's name on it and with me as custodian of the account. I asked after we signed if I would be able to see the account when I logged into my account online. The clerk assured me I would be able to see it. I needed an account in George's name to have his Social Security checks direct-deposited.

Anyway, we walked out with no paperwork, and I have yet to see the account on my page on the bank's website.

Thursday night was Hurricane Hermine. Our neighborhood, a manufactured home community, didn't have any problems. The wind was blowing strong much of the night.

Friday it was still raining on and off. The wind had stopped. I drove us to Anytime Fitness. Anytime Fitness was closed! Reason... no power. The power was out in parts of town.

We went next door to Winn Dixie. A clerk by the door told us we could only buy stuff off the shelf. All things from the coolers and freezers were being destroyed. The power went out at 2 a.m. It was now 9:30 a.m.

The Winn Dixie staff was gathered around shopping carts full of wrapped cheese and other items from the coolers. They were scanning them in and the scanner was saying "DESTROY, DESTROY." I felt like I was walking through the scene of a science fiction movie.

Back at home I worked on getting a handle on our financials with the unpaid bills and selling the two rental homes during our trip.

On Saturday mornings our Withlacoochee Bicycle Riders (WBR) group meets for breakfast at the Hen House in Inverness. We have been riding and dining with the WBR since we moved to Florida eight years ago.

I set the alarm so we would be up in time.

We had three flat tires among our two recumbent trikes when we arrived home from our trip. George had changed the tubes but not the tires. One of the tires of my trike must have still had something in the tire poking the tube because my front tire was flat again.

No problem; I have a two-wheel bike for such occasions.

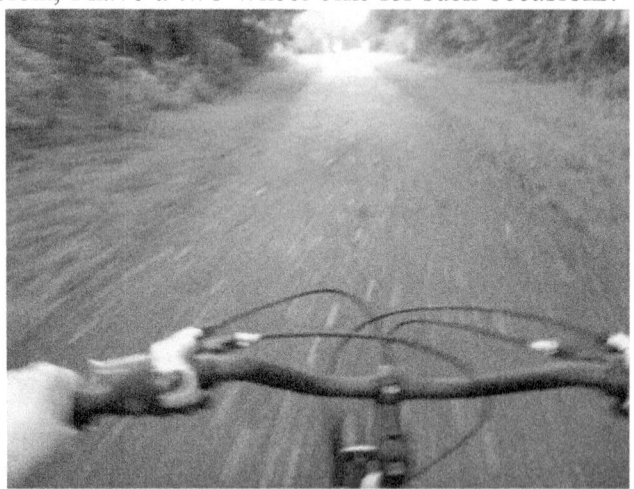

There was a lot of debris on the Withlacoochee Trail still from the storm.

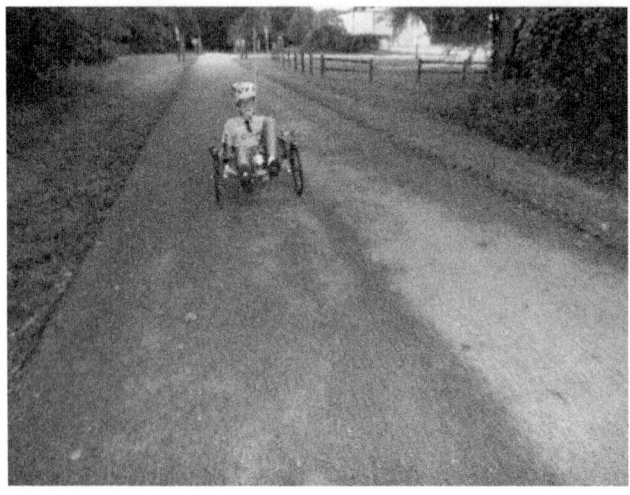

There were about 16 people at breakfast. *And*, one of our bike friends, Dick, bought our breakfast! He said he was glad to see us back safe.

Thank you!

At home, our neighbor Dianne came over and gave us three fruit from her cactus. She said the seeds are crunchy, and the fruit is slightly honey-sweet; it was good!

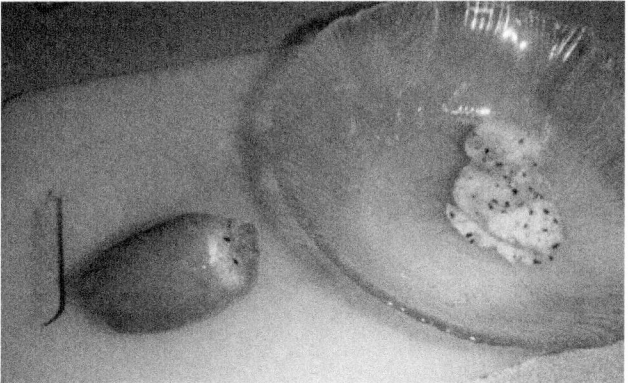

We got a call from our Canadian neighbors Louise and Richard. We do a lot with them in the winters and have gotten quite close in the few years we have known them. They told us they might not make it down this year.

I turned the phone over to George so he could say "Hi" and George started to cry. "I miss you guys," he said. Louise was surprised he was so emotional. The part of the brain that keeps that in check is gone. Plus he is dealing with having this dementia happen to him.

I got a call from my sister. We had a nice chat. I told her I had been thinking about looking for a duplex in the area. The lawyer had said to buy a big house because if George needs nursing home care it will take all our funds before we can start getting financial assistance from the government. They allow the well spouse to keep the house, a car, and a bit over $100,000.

Right now we live in a manufactured home on rented land. So that isn't much of an asset for me to keep if I should survive George. Anyway, I mentioned this to my sister. I was in the kitchen talking. George was in the living room reading.

After I hung up George came in and said, "So you are thinking about buying a duplex?" It surprised me. He's doing well today!

At around 2:30 I asked George if he wanted to go for a trike ride. Yes, he did. He had changed my tire; we were ready to roll.

As we rode, I started feeling better and better.

I started feeling really good and even did some sprints. George and I were both happy to be on this nice wide trail with shade and without having to stop and read the map.

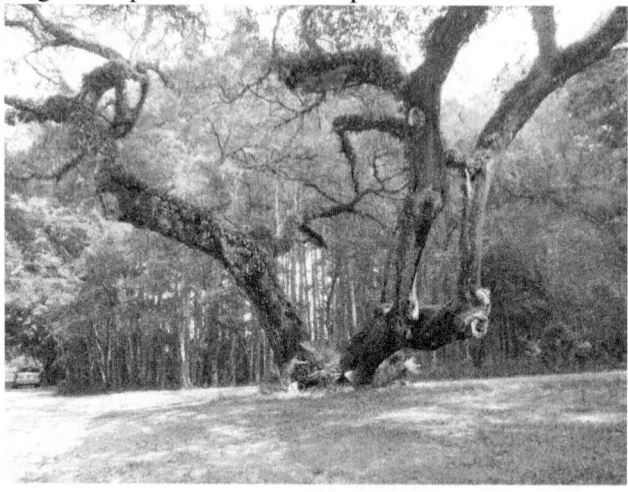

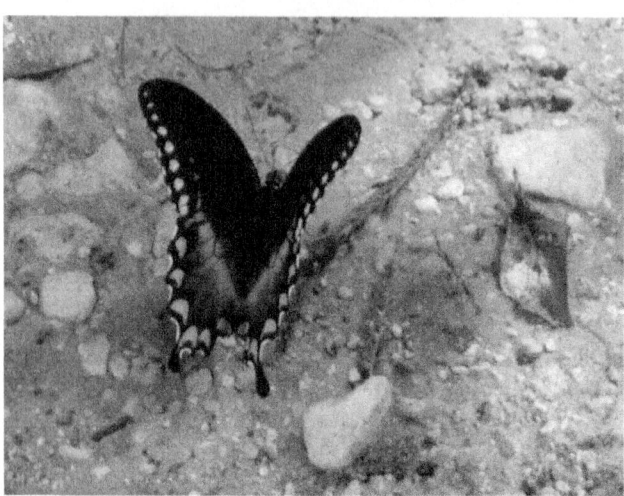

I asked George if he wanted to go into Nobleton and see if the ice cream shop was open. He smiled and said, "Sure!"

It was 4:00 on a Sunday and... it was open!

The owner dished out our ice cream and then told us we could go behind the shop and sit in the shade by the river....

Oh my! It was lovely!

We sat for a long time... as grey clouds rolled in with booming thunder.

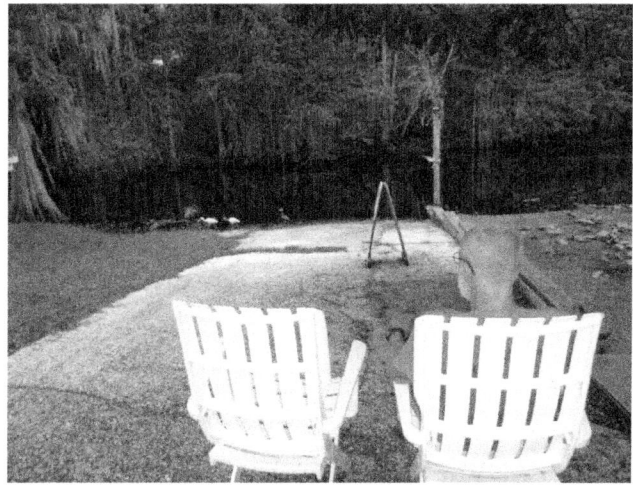

After a long sit we decided to head back. We could see the rain coming. We pulled over and stood in the doorway of the Nobleton Post Office waiting for the worst of it to pass.

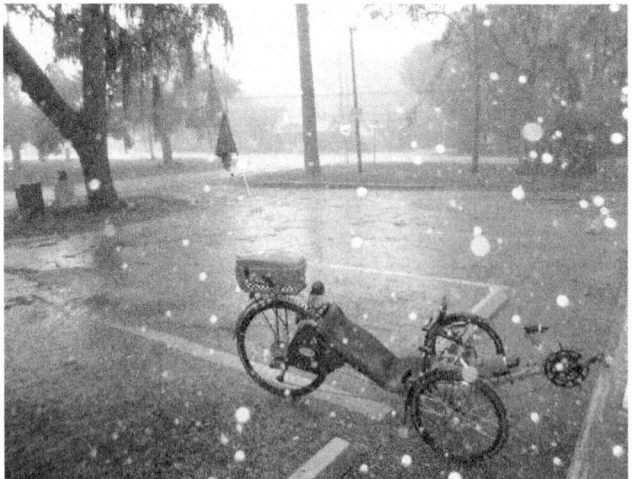

George used to complain and avoid the rain like it was acid or something. Now he says, "It's just water."

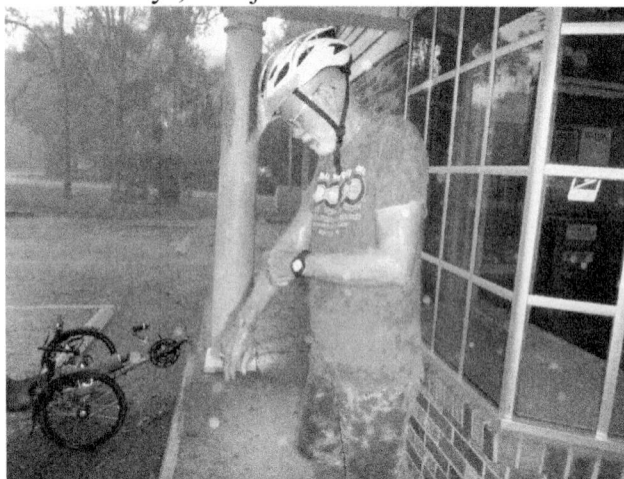

How wonderful to be on our trail, wide enough to ride side-by-side.

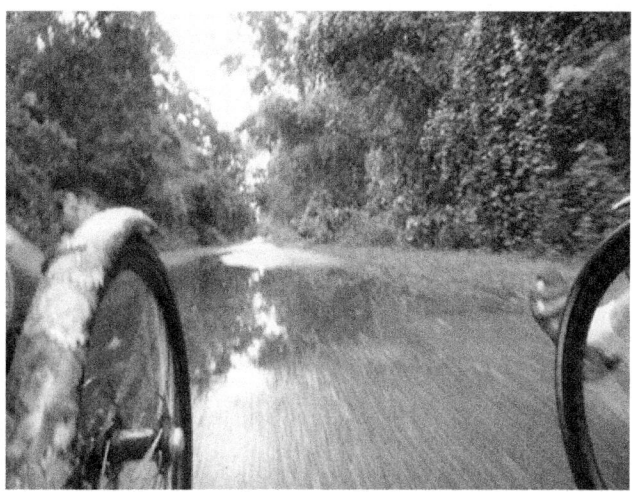

Monday morning I went for a walk before George was out of bed. I saw my neighbor Diane and walked with her a bit. I told her about needing to buy a house and she told me that she and her daughter are both nurses. They will help me when it is time. I don't have to put George in a home! She said we were much better off staying in this neighborhood where we have support.

I said, "When he starts wandering..." and then I realized that in this neighborhood people would know where he belonged. We have support here.

I am relieved and want to believe.

I signed up for a September 14th "Coping with Dementia" for caregivers. If I learn something new, I will share it with you.

Money Money

September 16, 2016

    I want to let you know that I have been making significant progress toward understanding where we are at financially and what we need to do moving forward.
    I have an appointment with Social Security the 26th.
    After that, on the same day, I have an appointment with a financial planner. That has forced me to list all assets and income for that meeting. With the information from Social Security, I will be ready to get a firm handle on stuff.
    I updated my résumé and now I am ready for a definite answer to the question, "Do I have to go back to work?" And "If so, full time or part time?" I have already sent my résumé a few places. I have not gotten serious enough to do what it takes, networking, asking, showing up....
    Part of me wants to go back to work. Work is good for us. I think that I really should work because I shouldn't be relying on the government to pay for care. Really, what kind of citizen am I?
    The other part of me thinks that maybe it is too late. There is no way to know how much longer George will be able to be by himself while I work. And all the money I make I will know that it will go into home care if not nursing care....
    We'll see if I get a resounding answer from the financial folks....

****

October 5, 2016

    I don't have a lot of answers to the questions I was pondering in my last blog post. I have made progress. Yet I still find myself wondering endlessly in thought circles.

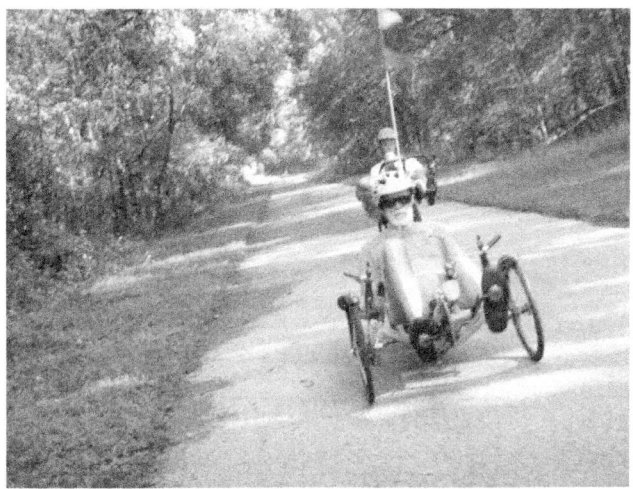

I am always watching for signs that the disease is progressing. In the meantime we continue to enjoy our trike rides and our friends.

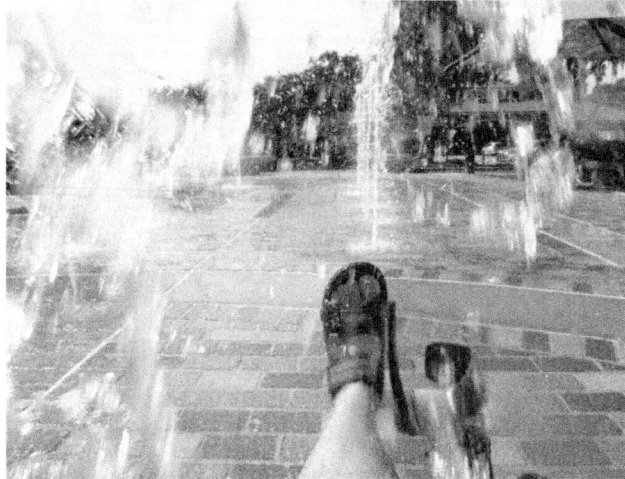

While I search for part-time jobs, George watches hours of *How It's Made* and *Bones*.

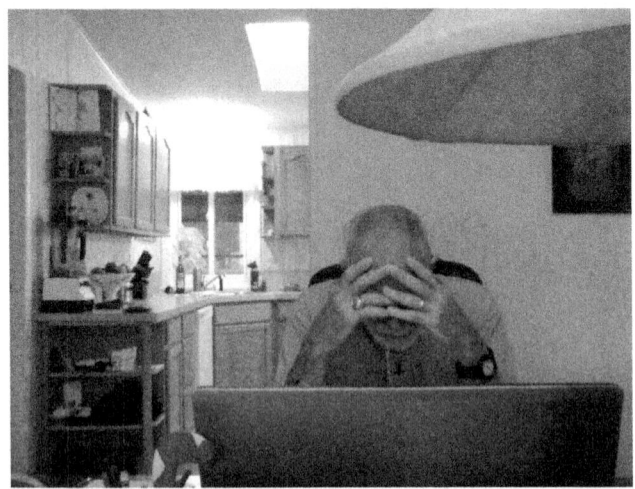

I discuss my concerns about my financial future with friends at our Saturday morning bicycle group's Hen House breakfast. One suggested a CPA she knew.

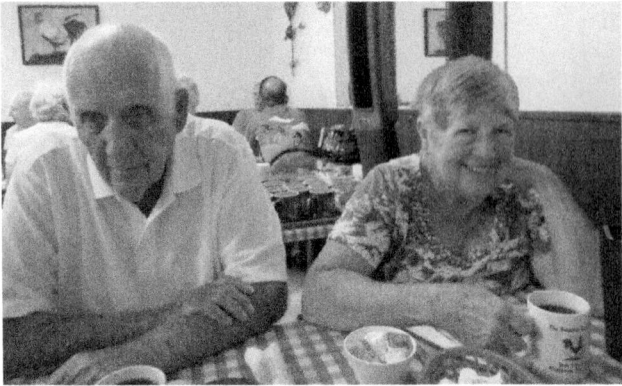

I made an appointment.

I thought George was doing well. He was making the bed, washing the dishes, bagging up the recycling. Then I stepped out back and found he had dumped a bunch of recycling on top of the brush. It was a soggy mess.

Every time I get up to take a walk after sitting a while, he jumps up and is ready to go with me.

I had an appointment with Social Security. Even if I wait until I am 70 to collect, my Social Security will be less than George's (we didn't think about this when deciding who would get the biggest paycheck at Rentapen, our business). My widow's social security will be a hundred dollars more than my own social security.

Withlacoochee bike friends told me about a home for sale within their HOA neighborhood near downtown Inverness. It is a kind of condo development right next to the bike trail. We went to look. The place, with windows only at the front and the back, was dark compared to our manufactured home that has three skylights.

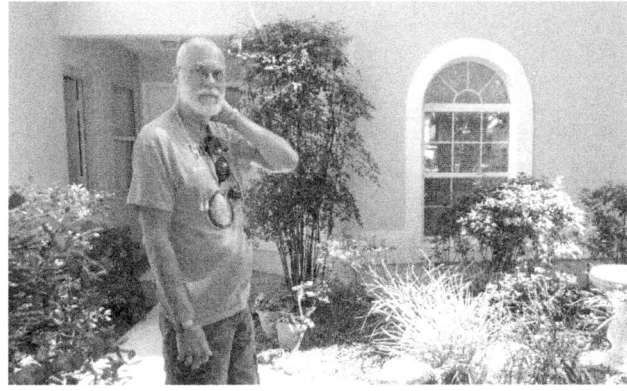

It is a big decision. I thought maybe the meeting with the CPA would give me some insight. I had sent him all our financial allocations and my goals and questions.

We met with him. He gets commission on insurance and refers to money managers. It would cost $2,500 to $4,000 for him to go through our stuff and give me some answers and advice. I took the information home to mull over.

I think about the cash I have sitting from the real estate sales I made while we were traveling. The money is waiting for me to make decisions. And I feel like a deer frozen in the headlights. I don't want to make a mistake... I can't *afford* to make any more stupid financial mistakes.

When I get home, I call a WBR friend who is a retired guy that used to do financial planning and at one time educated us about mutual funds. He recommended I call a "Fee-based certified financial planner." He said with George's diagnosis of progressive dementia, the prognosis is predictable. Long-term care is in his future, so we have to work with a planner that has elder planning skills.

I did call a CFP office. I left a message. In the meantime I sign myself and my friend Debra up for a class called "Women and Money."

The Withlacoochee State Trail had its fundraising ride. We ran the trailhead at Townsen Park which is about 14 miles south of Inverness.

We made lots of Tutoreos.
    Peanut butter on Oreos
    A slice of banana
    A raisin

Don't forget the raisin! George was the raisin man.

Our team had great fun with our Tutoreos, visiting with the bikers, and seeing the interesting bikes.

Hurricane Matthew

October 6, 2016 and October 7, 2016

Hurricane Matthew is heading north toward Florida. The Governor has declared the whole state should be prepared for this emergency.

After listening to seasoned Floridians, I learn that the eye of the storm isn't just the bad part. The storm causes other storms, so it is common for tornadoes to touch down.

I get offers from four couples to come stay with them during the storm. I am feeling the love!

Debra is going to be alone during the storm. I decide to go keep her company and get strong (brick vs. mobile home) shelter.

I go get three days' worth of non-cook food so we can tough it out if the electricity goes out.

I wrote up an offer for the condo we had looked at last week and we went over to see the place one more time and present the offer. He was pleased we were back, but not so pleased with the offer. He asked if we were "believers." He is very Bible-religious. I said, "We believe in our own way." When I presented the offer, he said he had to check with the other lady who had shown an interest. I gave him 24 hours to decide.

Back home, we put potted plants and other objects that might fly around in a big wind onto the screened porch. Then I started packing to go to Debra and Glen's to sit out the approaching hurricane. George stood by me in the kitchen as I packed, waiting, and a bag in his hand with his book and our sunglasses (his extent of what to pack). I am packing four days of water, four days of food, personal items, and flashlights.

I walk from the room. When I return, my stack of empty bags is gone from the kitchen counter, the bags I was going to fill. George had put them in the car. I asked him to go get them. He goes. He comes back with something else. I ask him again. He goes. He comes back empty-handed. Third time was a charm.

Not a good day... the excitement I suppose.

I tell him to get his cosmetic bag and cosmetics and don't forget your eye drops (glaucoma). He goes to the bathroom. He comes back with his eye drops and drops them in his bag of clothes. He's done. Uhhh. I hunt the drops out, go get his cosmetic bag and fill it with the essentials... toothbrush, deodorant, etc. Then he gets into it. He's got to have his vitamins and his large bottle of mouthwash and more.

I had asked him three times if he had packed a clean shirt. He said yes.

"Are you sure?"

"Yes, yes, yes."

When we arrived at my friends, I start unpacking the van, and on the floor of the van is a framed picture. It is a watercolor picture of him riding away on his orange trike on a winding path in a pine forest. George had painted this picture under the guidance of an artist and art instructor neighbor. This was his most precious item to save from the hurricane, I suppose.

This morning at our friends' I get up early. George is up shortly after in clean shorts and yesterday's shirt.

"Why didn't you put on a clean shirt?" I ask.

"No clean shirts," he says.

It is 7 a.m. and no wind yet. Wind picks up in Orlando at 8 a.m. this morning. We may see wind picking up about... 10? 11? Don't know.

I debate - should I drive home to get him shirts? Instead, we go for a walk.

Downsizing

The hurricane completely missed our area of the state. It skimmed the east coast.

While we were at Debra's during the day Hurricane Matthew was to hit, we got a call from the owner of the condo on which we had made an offer. He accepted our offer! We don't have a closing date. We have to wait and see if he gets accepted into the place he wants to move.

Part of our offer was to help him move the stuff he wants to take with him and handle whatever he leaves behind.

Right away, our friends Regis and Cindy offered to help us help him move. Debra offered help with packing up dishes and stuff. Our friends are wonderful!

We are expecting a call from the seller any day saying that he wants to move quickly.

Step-by-step I am looking at what we will move and what we should get rid of. I put some things on Craigslist for sale. I started a pile for the charity thrift store.

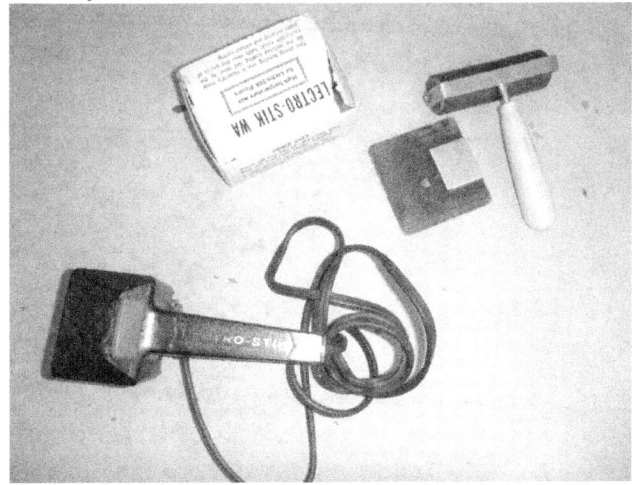

I studied electronics years ago. Solder wire and connectors are found in a drawer.

George worked many years ago as a pencil and paper engineer before computer-aided design and drafting were main-stream. We have an electric eraser and special brushes for sweeping the eraser crumbs off the paper.

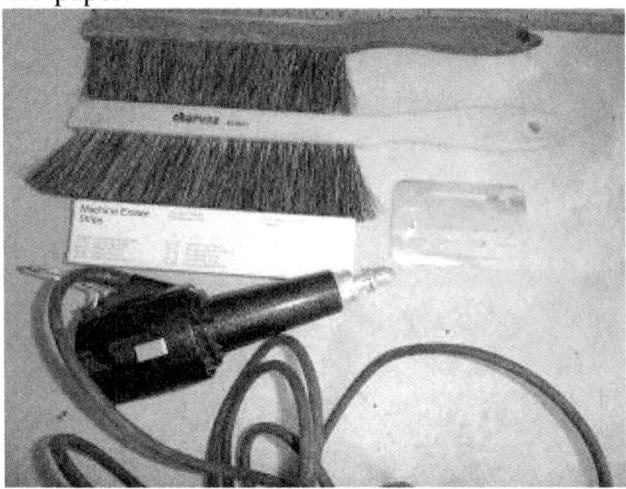

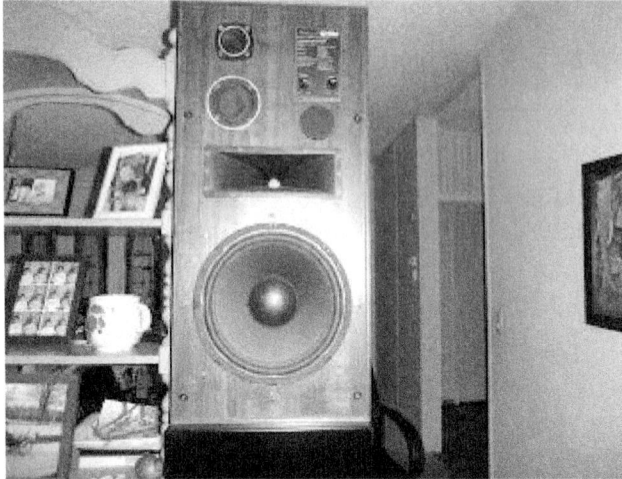

Our CD player and amp weren't working for a long time, so I decided to put the big speakers up for sale along with those electronic devices.

Today we finally got a buyer for the speakers. He is on his way. So I monkey with the CD player and amp trying to get them to work so I can show him how good the speakers sound.

Finally, I hit the right buttons. BAM! Great sound! George and I laugh and hug and dance... and then... oh my. George doesn't want to sell it now. It works! So I call the buyer three times and leave messages. I text him - no answer.

The buyer shows up. I dash out the door to greet them and I blurt out, "My husband has dementia, and I got things working so I could demonstrate the speakers work, but now my husband is crying because the music sounds so good, and now he doesn't want to sell them."

They understood though they were disappointed. I showed them some other things we had to sell and offered them for free, but he paid a bargain price for them instead. Fine, we still have the speakers.

Big heavy speakers to move, complex wires to hook up to the big heavy speakers and from amp to CD player - George says, "I can hook them up again, I know how." I don't say anything.

Today we have a memorial dinner to attend. I pick out George's clothes. When we are done getting dressed, George can't find his wallet. I know it is in the house. I try not to panic while flogging myself for not taking his credit cards out sooner and making copies of his other information.

We go to the memorial. George is smiling and crying at the same time. I don't know if it is hitting him that he is losing it because he lost his wallet or if he is emotional because he knows we are moving away from all these good neighbors. I don't ask. He probably doesn't know himself.

After the memorial we do a thorough search in the house. We don't search long when I find the wallet and keys in the pants he wore yesterday. No big deal. We go for a walk in the neighborhood. We stop to chat with a friend who just got a dog. Her husband has early stage dementia.

I have been thinking; a good way for me to make a little extra cash is to do pet sitting. The open door symptom of dementia is something I have to watch and solve first. We don't want to lose someone's pet! Next week we watch Regis and Cindy's two little dogs. I think we will be OK at this home. The only door George forgets to close is the one to the lanai, which has other doors.

I think I found a financial planner. I have my first meeting with him this coming Wednesday. This person is asking the right questions. He will advise and educate me, not take my money and manage it for me.

In the meantime I signed up for a women and money class and my friend Debra signed up too. The teacher is young and is talking about saving $25 a month for retirement. She went into debt for her car and talks about how she aims to have a great credit score. I am not impressed and have a hard time not laughing in class. All the students are older, either retired or close to it. So far she has only advised us to cut down our spending by writing everything down as we spend it.

Good idea... I only do it for one week. Then there were big money items: the inspection of the new house, a cap on one of George's teeth. I think, *There are always these big money items, why do I think this month is any different*? I do think that, and I get frustrated and I stop writing stuff down.

I chat with my Fidelity investment advisor who walks me through their program and tells me I will run out of money in 2035. She says, "You will need to go back to work." And, "The good news is you have time."

I meet with a job coach through a government funded program called Career Source. I start sending out résumés for part-time work. First I hit the health and fitness clubs. Might as well work in an environment I love and do something I love, right?

Today I put our house up for sale. I love our home. We love our home. I love the new purple shutters that George and I put up on the house yesterday. I love that our neighbors cheer when they see them. I love that our neighbors say they will miss us when we are gone. Some see the for-sale sign and stop by to chat.

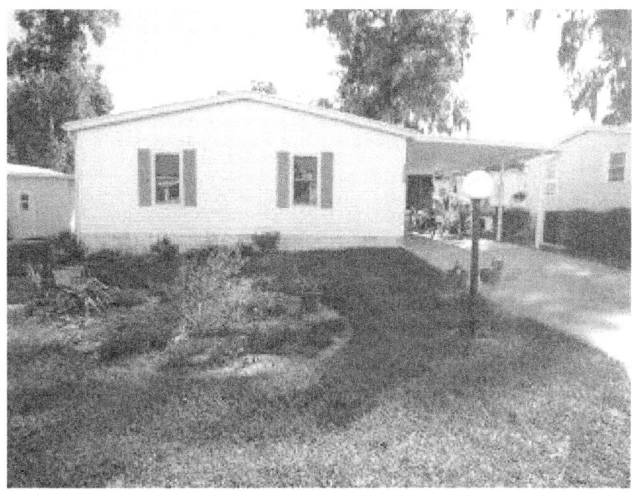

George had a birthday. We went to Debra's for dinner and she had birthday balloons up for him. We are so blessed with wonderful friends and neighbors. We are blessed with George's sweet nature.

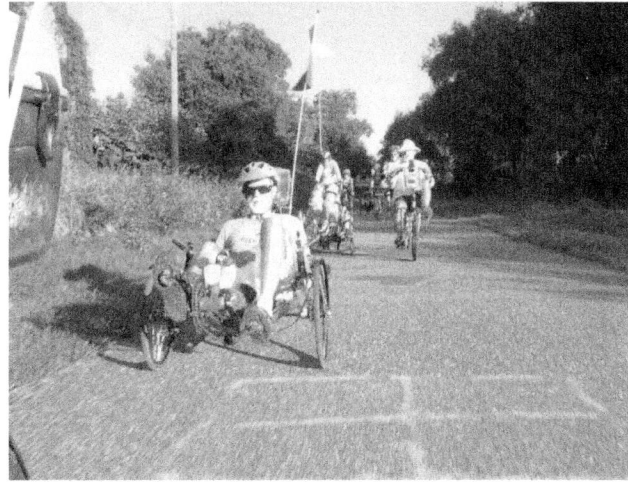

As I write this, we do not have a closing date on the new home we are buying. It is in a neighborhood with several other couples with whom we bike. It is adjacent to the Withlacoochee Trail so we will no longer have to cross a busy highway to get to it.

It will be a good move. The house will be one asset I can keep when or if George goes into a nursing home and we run out of funds to pay for it.

Fun While Living With Alzheimer's

January 22, 2017

Missing You!!
Even though we aren't traveling right now, we are still on a great journey...this wild ride living with dementia.
The fun times...

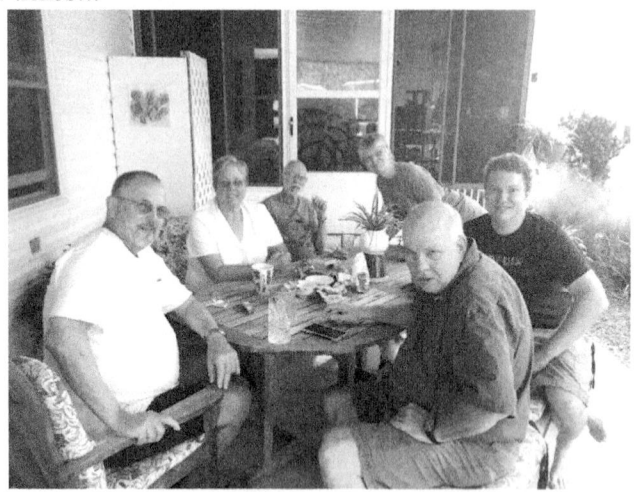

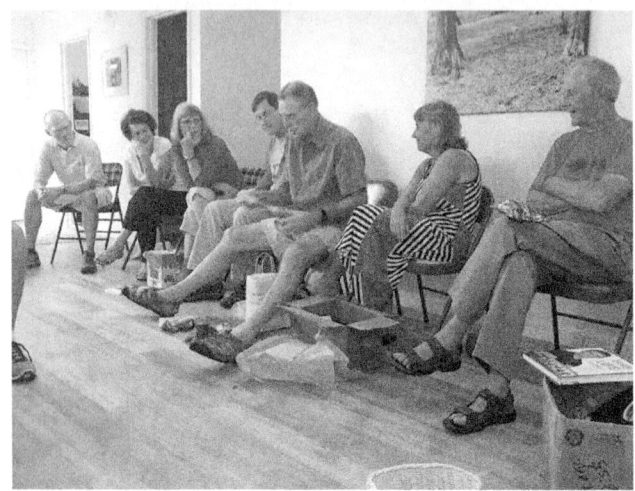

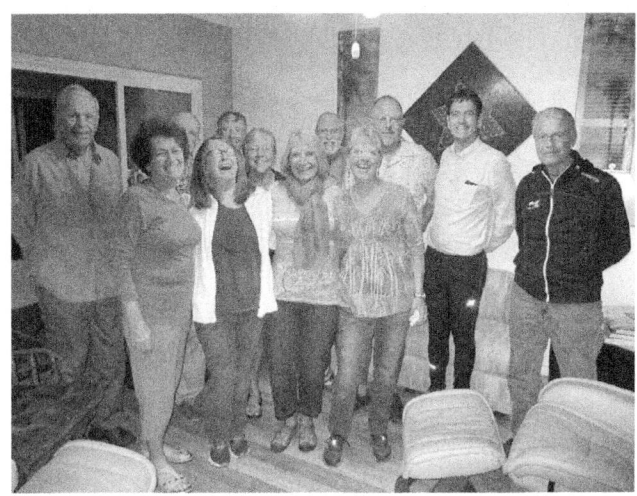

And the times when I try to remain calm, and I tell George (as he would have said before his brain started deteriorating) "It is what it is."

Right now it is January 2017 and our snowbird friends have arrived. I want to host lots of dinners and parties and gatherings. I want to attend lots of fun activities and go on long all-day rides. It is what we have done since we moved to Florida. But even with all the busy-ness....

I miss you.

I miss sharing the little things that happen day-to-day. I miss having each of you with me in those moments. I miss thinking how this moment looks from the *outside*.

I am afraid. I am afraid if I don't record these moments that they will be lost in the fog of my own memory which will fade someday too. I am afraid that when George passes I will be overwhelmed with guilt because I will only remember the times my patience came up short.

I won't remember all the good times, the laughs, the dances, and all the hugs.

Out of fear and nostalgia for the community you helped me create by following our 2016 journey, I will keep posting, keep updating, and keep this journal-thing going. At least try when I can pull myself away from the day-to-day.

First of all, let me update you on what has been happening since I last posted.

We moved! So many decisions and so much to do; no wonder I wasn't posting. I had to pick and contract for new flooring and painting. Manage to pull the funds together in time for closing.

And then there was the move itself. Our Withlacoochee biking friends helped a *lot*! Wow! Even the ones with bad backs helped in any way they could: carrying the small items; unpacking the dishes; sweeping the floors. Debra delivered lunch to us; Glen took George to run errands. Regis used his big van to haul stuff. Regis and Cindy returned to our old place to vacuum up all the pieces. We had probably 10 friends here! And I was supposed to be standing and telling them where to put stuff and not doing a very good job of it.

Then a few days later two more bike friends, Jerry and Dave, came over and put up pictures so perfectly. I love it!

You may be wondering how George is doing.

George seems happy. But he doesn't tell me so unless I ask. He still says "I love you."

And the other day, Friday, I couldn't believe it....

But before I get into what I couldn't believe on Friday, I first have to give you some background information.

I am working part-time at a little bike shop on the Withlacoochee Trail in Floral City (Trailside Bike, formerly known as Hampton's Edge). I started in late October, 2016.

Recently I started taking George with me when I go to work. It works out well right now because the owner is gone and George can sit in his office chair, see me, do his coloring and watch his videos (he has moved on from *How It's Made* to *The Three Stooges*.) He is very quiet and my co-workers are supportive.

I started taking him to work with me because one day... we were about ready to hop on our trikes and go meet the group for a ride. George went to use the 1/2 bath on the first floor. He was in there a long while; I was concerned.

I heard a flush and he opened the door, and I saw that the toilet was overflowing behind him. George stood by and watched as I turned off the water. I ran into the garage and got the plunger and some big rags to soak up the mess. George followed me every step... a few paces behind.

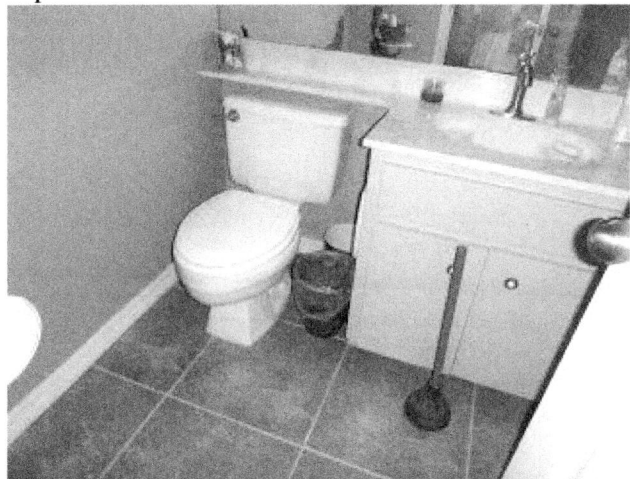

When I got back to the bathroom, I laid down the rags to start soaking. Both of us tried to get the plunger to work. It was the former owner's plunger and it didn't plunge. Fortunately, our neighbors (who also ride with the group) had not left yet. I borrowed their plunger.

The mess cleaned up, we got on our trikes and started down the road. Then I saw George sit up in his trike and reach to wipe something off his sock. It was POOP!

Let's just say my exclamation was appropriate to the situation.

We returned home. Before we entered, I directed him to take his shoes off because I saw they were full of poop too. Now there is poop on his fingers. I was yelling, "DON'T TOUCH THE WALLS!"

I got him cleaned up. As I washed him off I said, "No big deal. It is what it is." I think his embarrassment emotion is gone. He didn't seem affected.

Afterward we went on the ride and caught up with some of the group at a stopping point. We had a good rest of the day.

That episode sealed the decision to not leave George home alone. I started to take him to work with me. Can you imagine the mess if I had been gone that day?

A few more messy incidents and we have graduated from incontinence pads to the full pants.

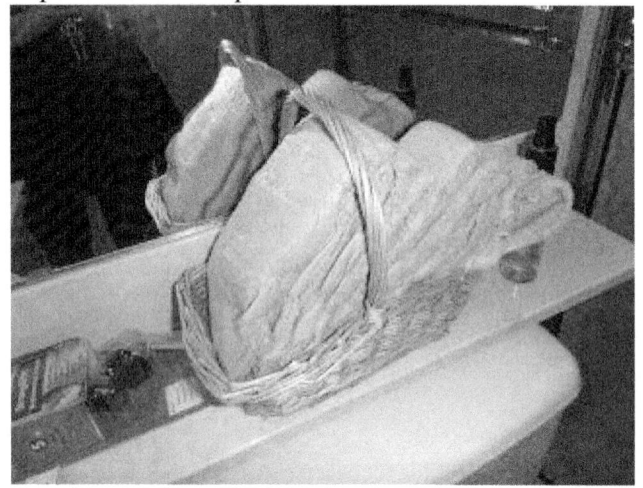

You never think of this, but a caregiver has to keep track. George is still cleaning and dressing himself most of the time. One thing he doesn't always do is change his pad. A caregiver at this stage must keep count. Watching the waste basket may not work because those with dementia may hide their soiled pants.

I am very fortunate in that George does not protest when I clean him up. He doesn't argue when I tell him to change his pad. So far... we'll see.

But to get back to the story I was going to tell you... the thing I couldn't believe....

On Friday, January 20th, he was with me at work.

At lunch time I took him outside to a picnic table. I ate my sandwich and left him at the table to finish his lunch. Right next to the bike shop is a flower shop. In all the years we have lived here he never stopped to buy me flowers. He even worked at the bike shop part time and he never bought me flowers. But that Friday...

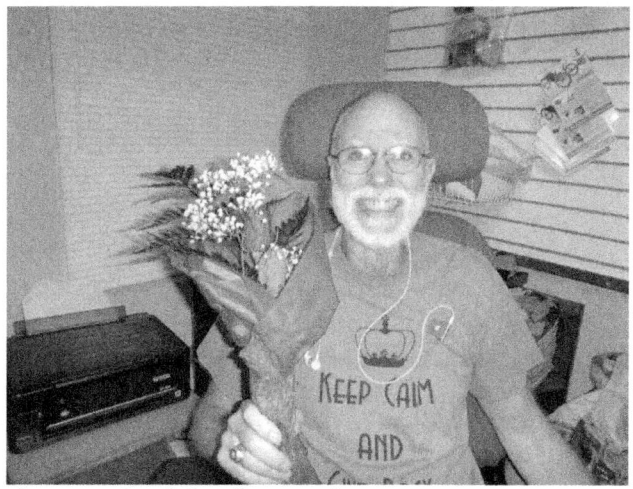

He must have noticed the flower shop....

Or maybe someone (a co-worker?) talked to him about it... I have my suspicions....

But then he has been... as a friend calls it... feeling "frisky." I can't imagine he could plot out a strategy for wooing me at this stage of his illness.

After work we rode our trikes from work to Inverness to meet up with a few friends. There was an old car show downtown and music to dance to. I showed the flowers to our friends and they took more pictures.

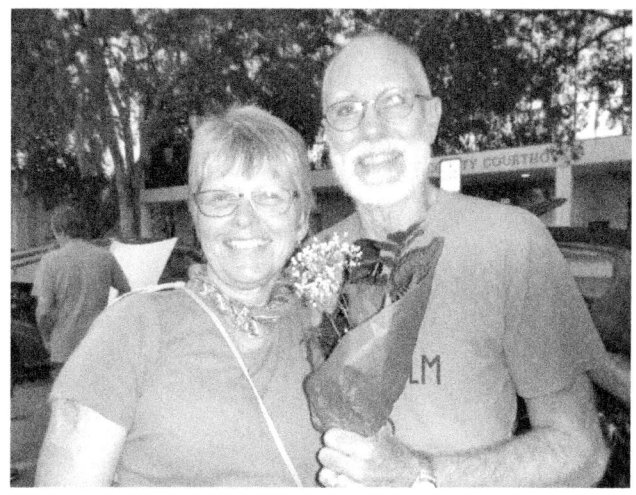

The music was good for dancing and George danced practically every dance with me/us... Frankie and I. The first dance we did was a line dance and George just followed me around the dance floor... not doing the steps, just following me around.

We had a great time.

I love that we are close to town. We both miss our old home and neighbors. Twice since we have moved we have gone back to our old neighborhood to walk around and visit folks.

One couple is on the same path as us. Learning as she goes she has shared information and experiences. She introduced me to the better support groups in the area. Another friend recommended the book *Alzheimer's Proofing your Home*, and so I ordered it from Amazon.

George and I joined the closest fitness club for a very reasonable fee. Mellodie's has character and is within walking distance. George does well; though his form sometimes worries me, he keeps going and has not injured himself yet.

Well, that is enough for now. I really should go sit with him and watch a movie or something. Tomorrow night I am hosting "Girls Game Night." I will probably set him up in the den. Our friend Bill gave us a used DVD player that is portable, like a small laptop. Maybe I will get him some movies to watch.

Trying to Maintain the Status Quo

This morning, I was wide awake by 4 a.m. Normally the early mornings had been my time to do things, catch up on correspondence, work and do yoga. I can still do all those things. But now I can do things that make noise because George gets up too. He used to need nine hours of sleep. Now whenever I go to bed, he goes to bed. Whenever I get up, he gets up. Even if I get up at 2 a.m. for a couple hours he is up with me. Me and my shadow....

Ladies Night

For Ladies Game Night I rented a couple movies from Redbox - things I thought George would enjoy. As soon as we got home from the store, he was fiddling with the DVD player. I explained to him, "No, those are for later when my friends come over for games. You can watch the movies then." He says, "Hee hee hee" and goes and sits down. Two minutes later I find him fiddling with the DVD again....

Then the ladies arrive, and I take him into the office and set up the computer and get a movie started.

George keeps coming out and standing over my shoulder. "The movie is not playing?" I ask. I set him up again. He keeps pushing buttons to stop the movie and comes out to get more food. He always needs more food. Each time, I get him more food and go back into the office and start the movie again and try to find the spot where he left off. He was able to tell me "I've seen that before" until we found a spot he had not seen.

Anyway, the gals said they had fun. And me? Well... I think next game night I won't be hosting or I will be sending George off to someplace else.

Traveling

Tuesday morning we packed up the van with our trikes and luggage. You know I packed. George can't pack anymore. I pack a bag; he picks it up and stands holding the bag waiting, waiting, waiting for me to finish packing the suitcases, the cooler, the beach bag, the trike stuff.

He helps me load up the trikes and helps haul a couple bags out to the car.

We were heading to Ormond Beach with our friends Debra and Glen. We had gone last year and had so much fun riding our trikes around and exploring the area. So Debra booked the same place for two nights. It is clean, comfortable, affordable, and convenient. We like the place.

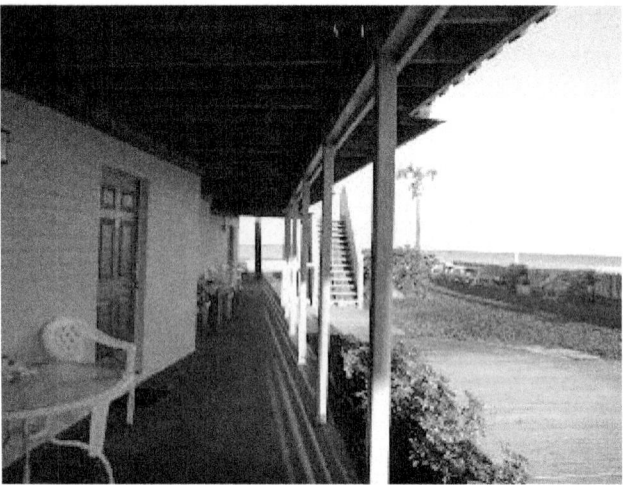

The drive is quiet. George doesn't talk.
At the motel we share a meal that Debra has cooked.
In our room, George surfs the channels just like he used to.

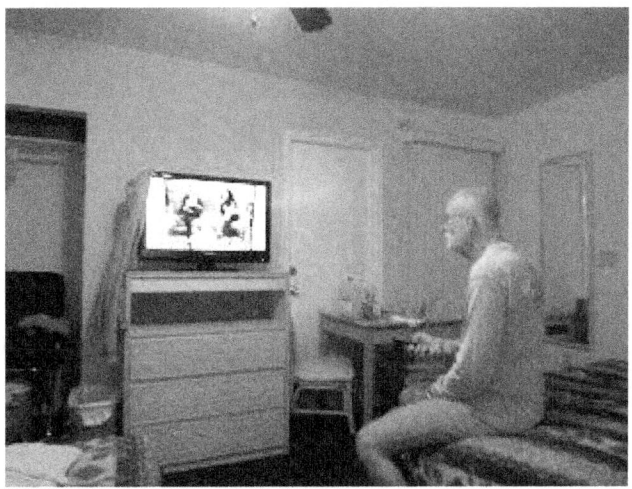

In the morning we walk along the beach. We are so early the sun has not even hinted it will be arriving soon. We stay out until it pops up over the horizon.

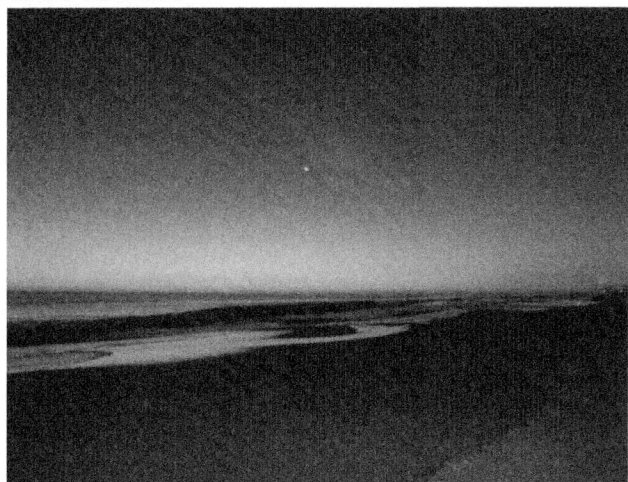

We go on two rides with Debra and Glen. We explore neighborhoods and boardwalks north and south of our motel.

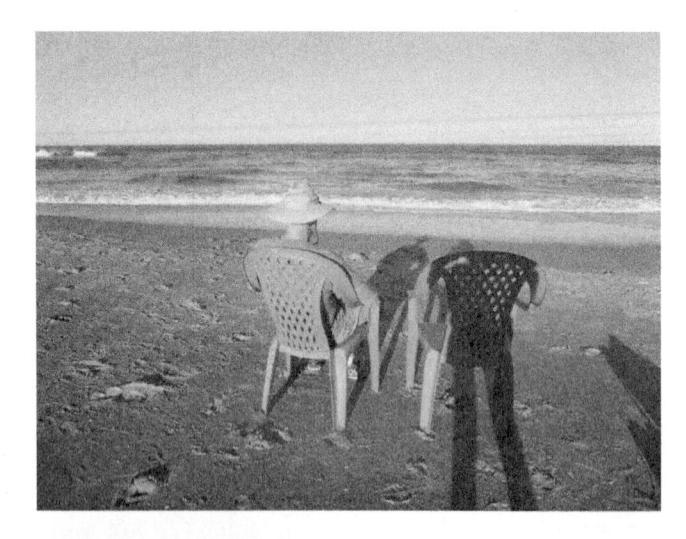

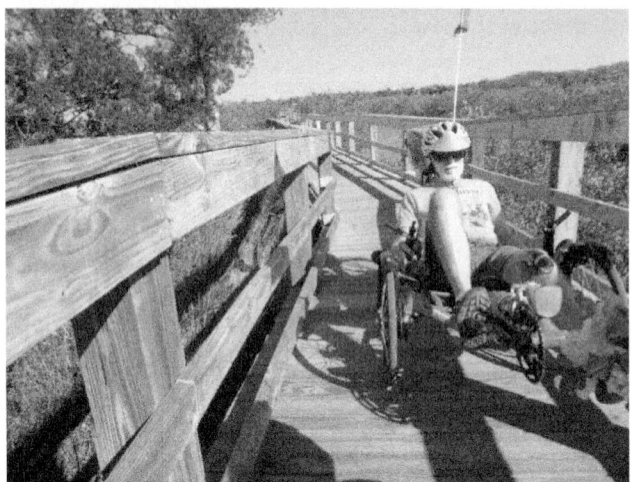

That night it was my turn to cook. I had a crockpot and had the stuff on all day while we biked. I thought it would be easy.

But George... first I had to clean up George and the bathroom. Then I would tell George to go sit at the table and one minute later he is standing back and eating the Fritos and sliced apples, etc.

I tell him to take dishes to the table and a minute later he is back in the room still holding the dishes. I take the dishes and him to the table and sit him down. I go back to our room to get more stuff ready. He is back in the room with me. When I put some food on the table he stays at the table. The thing is I have brought just enough for the four of us. Not enough for a compulsive eater. And I get a bit sharp with him when he continues to reach for food.

Debra tells me to relax.

I finally get the meal on the table and I feel inadequate because I didn't plan for more food, but just getting packed and out of the house was a feat. I tell myself not to be so hard on myself, but I am embarrassed, even with good friends.

The stay was only for two nights. In the morning I just wanted to be home.

We got back home in time for an appointment that I had forgotten about. Whew!

I had offered to visit with a friend who had knee surgery and whose husband has dementia. I offered to take her to dinner. I was glad I got home in time to go.

We took them to a restaurant. George got fish and chips. His previous self was a strict vegetarian. Some day ahead he will be eating burgers and bacon.

Dementia Caregivers Stuff Feelings

March 1, 2017

Sigh...
Now our life is all about drudgery (just kidding).

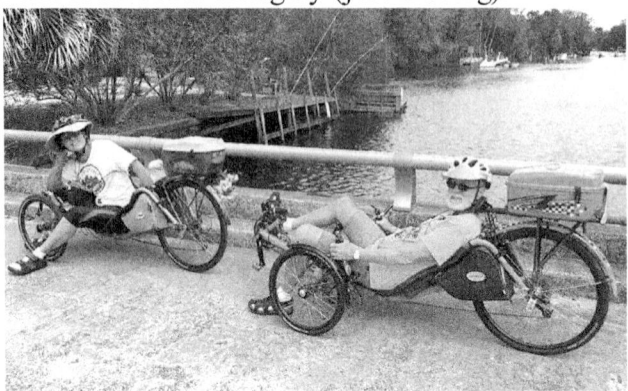

We bike, we dine with friends, and this past Thursday we went to The Villages with some friends and danced the night away.

This is us as we were leaving for The Villages.

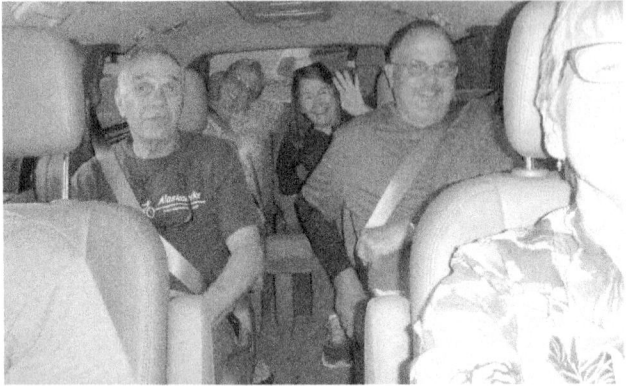

If you don't know what The Villages is, it is a retirement community with manicured lawns and three downtown areas with music on the square every night of the week. It is about 30 to 45 minutes away from where we live.

The band we went to see was The 45s. They do a lot of good dancing songs.

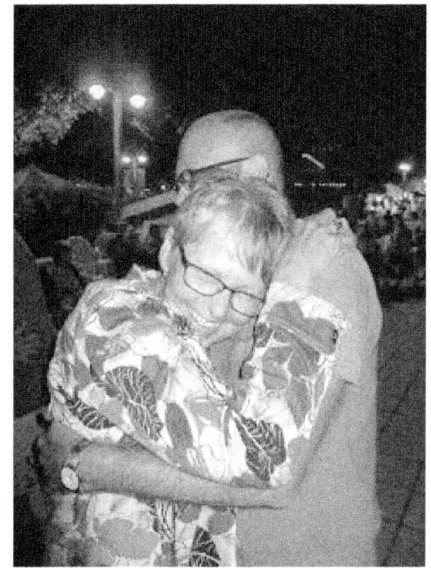

They played *Nights in White Satin* a song that was popular when we were dating. George sang as we danced - off key... very off key. We were laughing together as we danced.

I was surprised at how much George wanted to dance that night. Even the fast dances. I could tell he was trying to match my step, so I had to keep it simple when we danced together. I kind of selfishly resented having to tone it down for him. I wanted so to just let go....

We had a great time. Our friends have continued to include us in their invitations and dinner parties.

So don't think it is all about poop and over flowing toilets and silence....

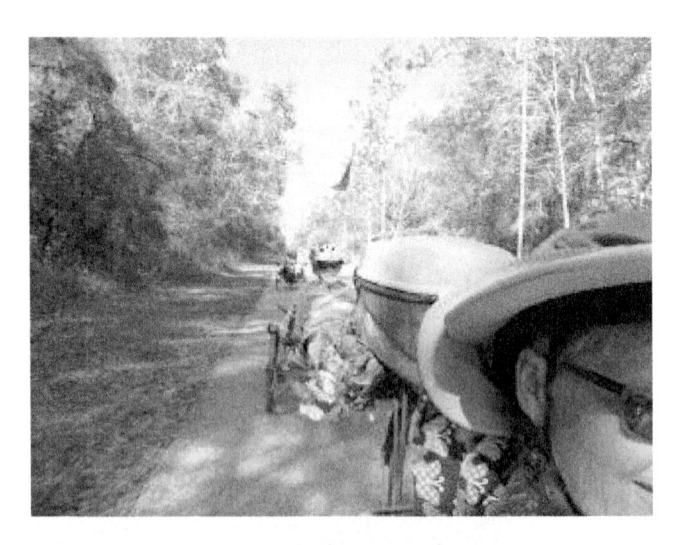

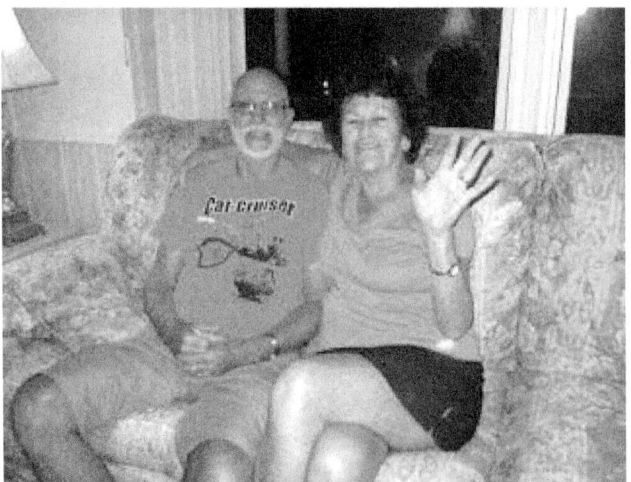

What is constant is that the George I knew is gone and I am feeling like I should be grieving more. There should be more tears. Mostly, though, I just stuff the feelings when they come, because there is work to do.

It is constant, it seems. That inner dialog to remain calm and kind… it saps energy. I want to lie down and take a nap, but then what would happen while I wasn't paying attention?

Do you have any pet peeves? Like litter or leaving the water running or leaving the refrigerator door open or sloppy eating or running the dishwasher when it is 1/4 full?

I just didn't realize how many little things get my blood pressure to rise.

There are the added expenses that no one plans for - the extra laundry, the compulsive eating. I try not to complain when he leaves the door open on cold mornings.

Well, when you are a caregiver to someone you love, there is no room for being particular. I am forever stuffing. Trying to be rational and kind when I want to make comments, provide instructions, and yell. Reactions are automatic waves that crash down on me and I have to keep still inside or at least, on the outside appear calm. Maybe this is a crash course in Zen or watchful meditation. I am watching my emotions without acting on them.

Yesterday on our regular Tuesday ride, we were almost home. We stopped in Hernando at the restroom. I had to help George out of the trike; he didn't have the right method (aim forward) and he didn't have enough strength... his arms shaking as he tries to lift himself using his assist bars.

I sit on my trike relaxing and waiting while he is in the bathroom. Then it gets a bit long... I wait some more... oh oh....

I knock on the restroom door. "You need some help?" I ask.

"Yes," he says. There is a pile of poopy tissue in the toilet. "Don't flush I tell him, it will overflow."

I go back to my bike and get the clean diaper and the handy wipes and the clean shorts. I am feeling pretty proud... a competent caregiver I am.

The poop is squashed on his butt (he must have messed before getting off the trike) and the tiny handy wipes aren't adequate.

"Note to self: next time pack a washrag."

Fortunately, this bathroom has running water. I start to work on the toilet, trying to flush only some of the paper at a time so it doesn't clog and overflow. Yes... that means grabbing some of the dirty tissue. I am breathing through my mouth.

The toilet flushes clean. Yeah! Success! I cheer and George giggles.

Then I use the toilet water to swish out the handy wipes after each wipe. Just like swishing those cloth baby diapers... remember? George is very cooperative and stands still and lets me wipe him down including his legs, his socks.

Finally he is clean. I bag up his dirty shorts and we toss the dirty diaper in the trash outside. There is even soap in the bathroom. We scrub our hands.

Back out by our trikes I raise my arms and cheer. "Yay! We did it!" I say, and George smiles big.

****

This morning we walk fast to the gym. I notice that if I am in front of him he walks fast with me, but if I am at his side he slows down.

After the gym we go to our neighborhood clubhouse and do yoga.

It is a lovely day. I check my phone. My friend Debra has texted me offering to take George for a couple hours this afternoon. I have plans, though.

Medicaid is calling at 10 a.m. to interview me for providing help and respite care. Then I have to go to the Key Training Center (15 miles away). They are going to provide one day of day care each week and I need to go there to sign some papers. Then I have to drive to Ocala to the eye doctor and get some paperwork and take that paperwork to the VA in Lecanto.

While I am getting some information together, I notice that George has gone into the bathroom and is in there a long time.

Uh oh....

This time I walk into the master bathroom, and George is standing in an inch of water without his shoes on. The toilet is flowing over the rim and George is holding a plunger and trying to take his socks off.

"OH NOOOO, OH NO, OH MY GOODNESS!" I exclaim as I reach down and turn off the water.

"George, you have to tell me when the toilet overflows! Why didn't you call me?"

George says nothing. George doesn't think to talk.

I plunge the toilet. George just stands there. "Go get the whole bucket of rags from the garage. They are next to the dryer," I say. "Hurry," I say.

I walk out and I see there is about a foot of soaked carpet in our bedroom. I reach for towels. I am so worried that the woodwork will get soaked and start puffing... ruined particleboard.

"OH NO, OH NO," I am still moaning. I take towels and lay them on the floor. Instantly they are soaked, and I pick them up and plop them into the shower stall. It is a lot of water.

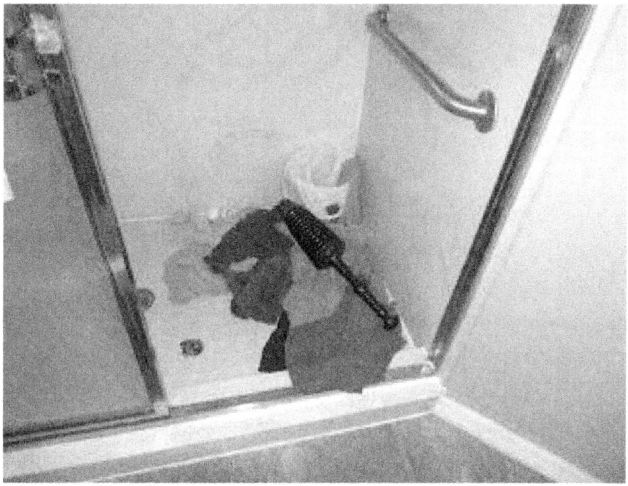

George returns holding two half towels.

I send him back for the whole bucket of rags. He returns with one more towel.

I send him back again: "Bring me the whole bucket." I am now wringing the towels and laying them down again to soak up more.

I am thinking that I am going to have to buy a wet-vac for such occasions... this is the third incident since January. Then I remember we have a carpet cleaner. It sucks up water!

George returns with the bucket of rags. Now I send George out to get the carpet cleaner from the garage as I still continue squeezing out towels and then laying them back on the floor. SOOO MUCH WATER!

He returns with the carpet cleaner. It is missing two containers... I go get them myself.

I vacuum and vacuum and vacuum the carpet by the door, and still more water comes up. We have to empty the receiving bucket three times, and still we are getting more water.

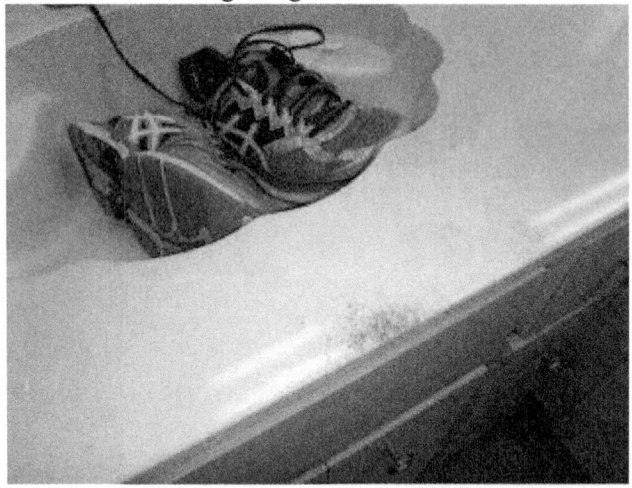

George vacuums while I finish up cleaning the bathroom. His shoes are soaked. I put them in the sink and notice a smudge of pooh on the counter. He can't stand up when he removes his shoes or his pants. He has to lean on something or sit down.

I clean off the counter and think to myself that I will need to buy a bed cover because he often sits on the bed to take his shoes off. Our beautiful quilt would be hard to clean.

We are almost done cleaning when I look at my watch. Almost 10 a.m. and time for my phone call.

While I am talking with the gal from Elder Options on the phone I am wondering what George is doing.

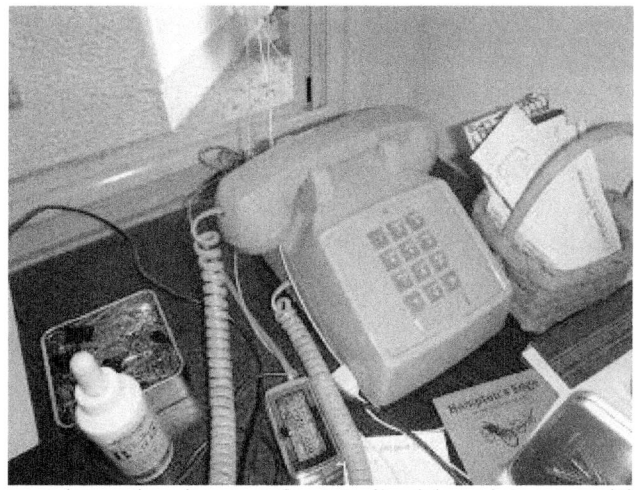

The woman interviewing me for Medicaid assistance with respite care and other help said the help will cost me about $160 a month. After I got off the phone I remembered I forgot to include a note we hold on the business in the assets I listed for her. So I called her back and left a message. The price per month will probably be higher. But still, $160 for a few days of respite and some help with meals and cleaning would be nice!

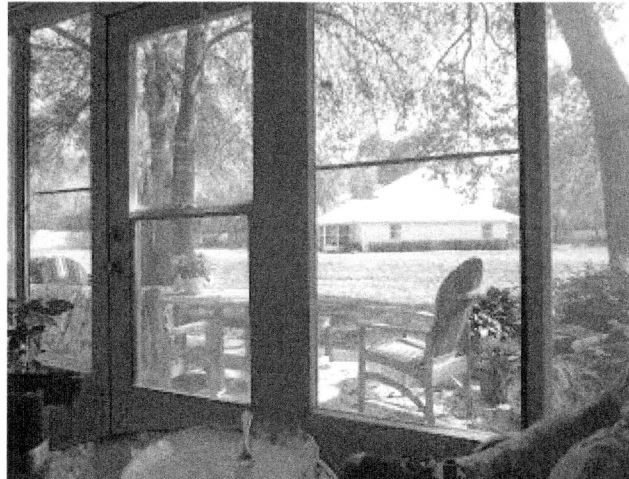

After the hectic morning I fixed us lunch and we sat out on the patio. George is dropping parts of his salad every few forkfuls and picking it up off the floor and eating it. I stare out at the beauty and try to find my happy place.

I think George's brain is now stuck in a loop. "What is Sue doing?... Where is Sue?"

This evening after supper I told him to go brush his teeth and I went to the kitchen. He went to brush his teeth. Then he came out and walked toward me still swishing his mouthwash. He then goes into the 1/2 bath and spits into the sink. I finish what I am doing in the kitchen and I go into the bathroom to brush my teeth. George follows me and pulls his wet toothbrush out of the drawer. It's dripping.

"What are you doing?" I ask.

"Brushing my teeth," he replies.

"You already did," I tell him.

He seems to doubt me a moment and then smiles and puts his brush away.

Next time you are cleaning the house notice how often you turn around. Then imagine having someone there two feet behind you. I have become so aware of how many times I walk into a room, stop, and turn around. He's always in my return path.

When I am working in the office on the computer I have learned to take the time to set him up in a chair with a movie or a game on his computer.

Tonight I got a call from George's friend Glen. He has a movie and would like to come over and watch it with George. Good news! I will finish this blog post and go for a walk... without my shadow! Thank you, Glen!

The Art of Dealing With Bullies

March 13, 2017

Yesterday was a "two poop day." I am getting pretty matter of fact about the clean-up.

This morning he was laughing a lot while watching the Three Stooges.

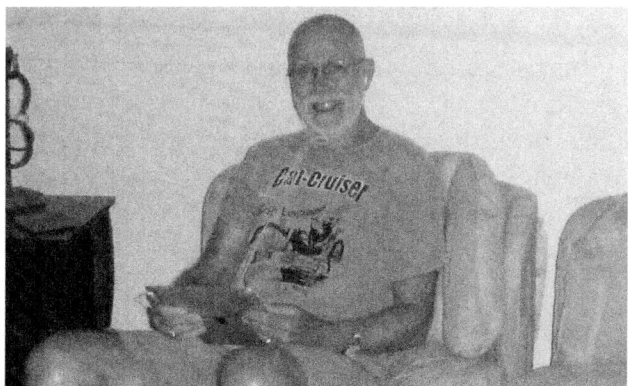

We went to yoga at the neighborhood clubhouse and then walked to the gym and....

The Bully Encounter

George likes to watch stuff. In the early stages of his illness, if someone glanced his way while he was watching them, he would glance away like he wasn't really staring at them. But that isn't the case any longer.

Today at the gym he was on a machine and watching this testosterone pumping guy. And the guy turned around and told him not to stare. George didn't comprehend and just smiled and nodded like people do when they don't really understand someone. The guy said, "I am serious! Stop it!" And George just smiled some more and nodded.

I went to the guy and said quietly, "He has dementia, go easy on him." And the guy commanded, "Then you got to get control of him."

I went over and explained to George he was to watch me, not the guy. But he watched me for only a little while and then was smiling and staring at the guy again. The guy said, "I can't lift with you staring at me, stop it. I am not kidding!"

I went to George and moved him to a different station with his back to the muscle guy. Then I went to the muscle guy and I said, "My husband is working with half a brain, but it is still bigger than yours. And his heart is twice the size of yours." No apology from him, just more whining.

I couldn't hang around; I was fighting off tears. I cried on the way home, walking in front of George as I do these days because if I walk next to him he slows down and stumbles more. George didn't see me crying.

I know the guy was on too much testosterone to think straight, but still, it really hit me how I am the mama bear now, protecting this... child.

Pooh Goo

A friend who is caring for her husband with dementia said she is going to the Alzheimer's support group this week. I asked her to ask a question for me, but I don't know if she will.

I said, "Ask if there are any pointers for getting poop off of hairy butts."

I am trying to figure out a better method. If I put him in the shower, then I have to dry down and clean the shower and clean up the chunks if there are any. The handy wipes do nothing but slide over the surface of the poop. I could go through a whole box of wipes in one clean-up.

So far a washrag and a lot of rinses work best. I hate rinsing little chunks of poop down the same sink I use for brushing my teeth. Yesterday while I was rinsing the rag for another go at the pooh, I knocked my toothbrush I had left on the counter and it fell into the sink. EWWWWW!!!!

I had a good laugh.

Yesterday I searched on the internet and found a bidet addition to the toilet. Tushy it is called. I emailed them to see if it takes chunks off hairy bottoms... how wide is the spray... I wonder if they will respond.

Day Care

George is taking well to Day Care at the Key Training Center in Lecanto. When I dropped him off on Friday he said, "They offered me a job here."

I said, "They did? Are you going to take it?"

He said, "I think I will."

"Good!" And I let the staff know they could put him to work when we arrived. I don't know if they did. When I picked George up that afternoon he said they had him color all day. That was his work. He seemed pretty proud.

Airbnb

As I reported earlier in this blog, I bought a bigger house on the advice of the elder attorney. We moved in on December 9, 2016 with the help of many great friends.

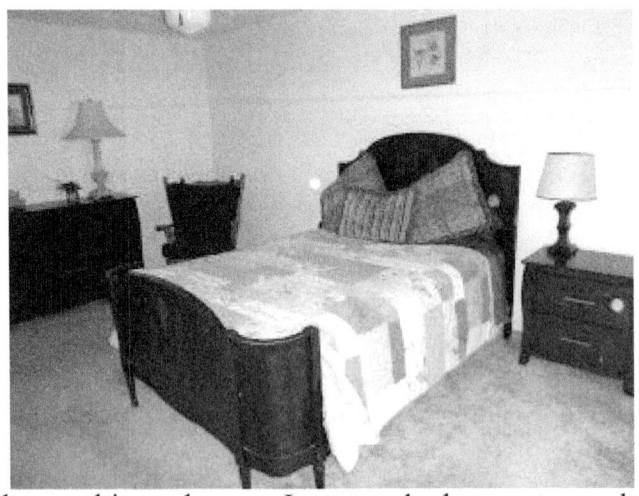

Now I have a bigger house. I put two bedrooms to work. I have a low price and it is high season in Florida, so March has been very good for renting the rooms. We are used to having people come stay with us because we have hosted bicycle tourists for many years through the website www.warmshowers.com.

Then I re-read the info on the HOA rules. I had already opened my big mouth and shared what I was doing with several people in the neighborhood. Now my neighbors know what I am doing. I had to quit. So much for that extra income stream! After March, there are no new bookings.

Friends Help

David and Jennifer, WBR friends of ours, came over and watched movies with George so I could get out by myself last week. Also Glen came and took George to a movie so I could go for a walk by myself. That was very nice. George can't walk as far; when we go too far he starts to lean and wobble.

Richard came over and re-hung a rack for hanging our hats and sweatshirts.

Every day I am grateful to have the support that we have. If you don't live close to us and want to be of help, go find someone close. Sit with someone so the caregiver can get some away time. Or offer to help with repairs and maintenance, drop off a meal, or stop by just to visit. The caregiver might be feeling isolated. Friendship is a wonderful gift!

Offer, and if they refuse, offer again and again. Adults are independent folks. We like to think we are handling things well, that we can do without assistance. But my friends have persisted, and I am so thankful for that!

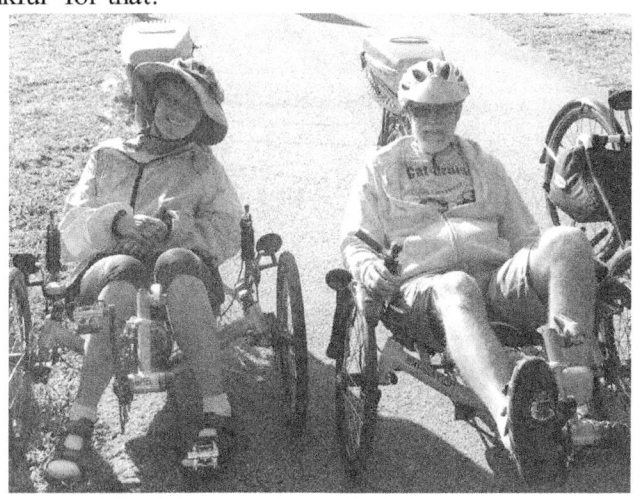

In-Home Help is Coming

We are now on the waiting list for getting some in-home help. When we do get the help, it will be respite care, meals, and house cleaning.

Shazammm!!

I was also wondering why I had signed up George for VA care when the insurance advisor told me to hang on to his Medicare and gap insurance given his diagnosis.

But I got a call from the VA social worker who agreed with that advice. VA is *on top of* your regular insurance. Get a physical from both each year to stay in their systems. Doesn't that seem redundant and wasteful?

The VA will send help for a couple hours twice a month for a year. I think I told them not yet; I will need it more later on.

That's the update for now.

It's Good, It's Bad, It Just Is

Thursday, April 4, 2017

"Do you want a fish sandwich?" I ask George.
He nods yes and says, "Fish sandwich."
"I think I will have the grilled cheese," I tell him.

We are out on the patio at the Riverside Cafe or Bar and Grill in Nobleton, FL, with our friend Glen. Next to George on the patio is a black lab/pit bull with a limp and a broken toe. He is kind of dirty; none of us reach to pet him.

The owner of the restaurant is also limping. She is in sandals with two middle toes on her left foot taped together and black and blue. She is working to remove paving blocks from a flat-bed trailer. She and a man (her husband?) are walking back and forth to the trailer, stacking the pavers on the ground by an outdoor stage.

It was threatening rain when we launched our ride today with the Withlacoochee Riders.

We usually ride north on Tuesdays, but a storm was passing through just north of us.

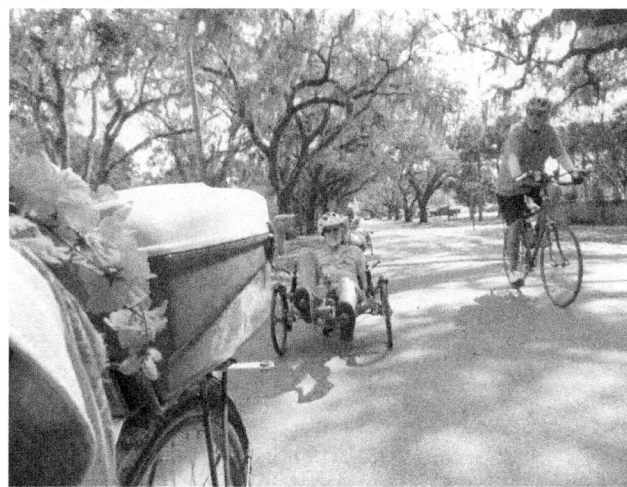

Just four of us took a chance and started biking south on the Withlacoochee State Trail.

So far the rain had not caught up with us and now it was just three of us sitting at the table at the Riverside Restaurant.

Glen and I talk about the menu and the paving project.

"What are you having?" George asks.

"I am having a grilled cheese," I tell him.

"Me too," he says and smiles at me his goofy lost smile.

"I thought you were going to have the fish sandwich," I say.

George smiles, nods and says, "Fish sandwich."

Until we order, the conversation with Glen is interspersed with a rerun of the fish-sandwich conversation with George.

I order for George and myself and after that, George no longer asks. I overhear the owner and the guy telling some other customers that the dog got hit by a car right there. I got the impression it happened a while back and that they were concerned that the dog had returned and the dog might get hit again. They must have called the owner because pretty soon a woman pulls up in a little grey car, greets the owner, pets the dog, puts the dog in her car, and drives off.

George eats the fish and leaves the bread. That is good. He has gained 17 lbs. since his diagnosis. He doesn't register "full." He gets hungry often. When we go to parties where the food is sitting out, he continually eats.

After we leave the restaurant the rain catches up with us. I pull out George's poncho and help him put it on.

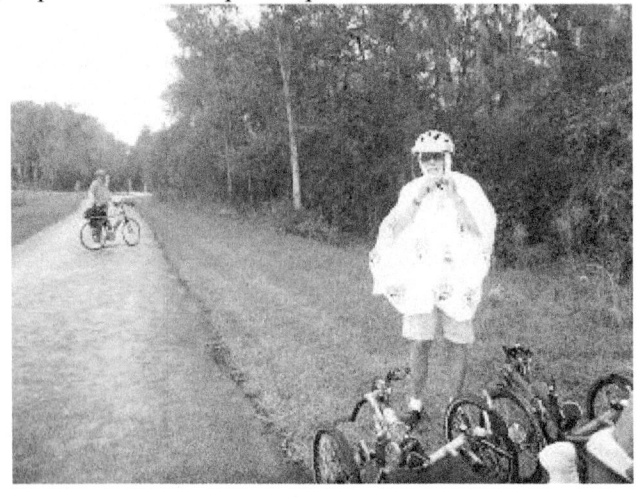

When we reach Floral City, George pulls into Trailside.bike. I get off my trike and go stand in front of him as he is getting off his trike.

"George, are you having trouble with your trike?" I ask.

"No." he says.

"Why did you stop here?" I ask.

He stutters and stumbles and chuckles nervously because he can't find the words or the reason. Finally he says, "I am going to get a new one."

"A new what?" I ask and wait as he struggles.

"A new bike," he says.

"A new trike?" I ask.

He nods.

"No, we aren't buying you a new trike. How would you like some new tires?"

His tires were worn and I had planned on getting some anyway. We buy new tires.

Glen offered to put them on George's trike for us. *Yes*! Now we have to find a time when our schedules and energy coincide.

Education

Tomorrow I start a seven-week course offered in Citrus County called SAVVY Caregivers of those with dementia. I am going to learn about communication, drugs (not for me, unfortunately), services, and stages of the illness.

I learned about it from the manager of the Key Day Care where I take George once a week. I normally take George on Fridays when I go to work at the bike shop. But for the next seven weeks I am taking him on Wednesday, and I will take George to work with me on Fridays. We will see how that goes.

Blessed With Good Friends

Our WBR bike friends Jennifer and David have been coming over once a week to watch movies with George. They take him for short walks and even fix him supper! While they are with him, I get to go somewhere. I can go for a walk or meet up with friends. Glen also comes over to watch movies and offers to have me drop George off to work on bikes with Glen in his garage. Debra has us over for dinner often.

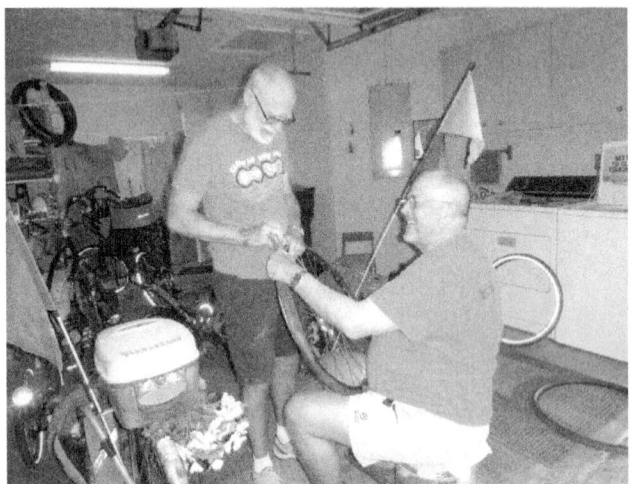

WBR friends Richard and Louise and Jerry have come to help fix things around the house.

This week, while WBR friends were with George, other bike friends, Mary Ann and Dianne, arranged to take me on their lake kayaking to relax. I arrived and they were down by the lake all ready for me. Wow. I am unbelievably blessed with good friends.

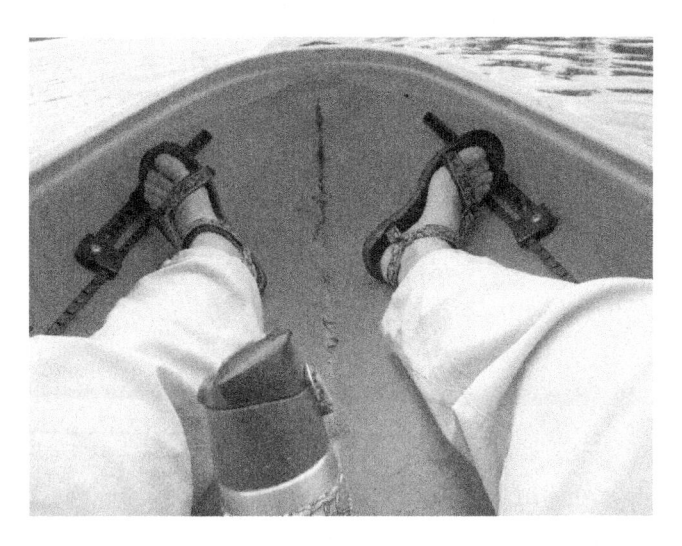

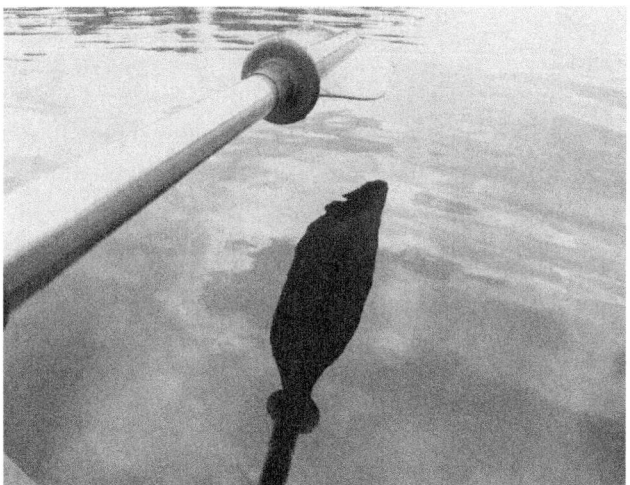

We saw beautiful cypress and lots of limpkins. After our kayak ride we still had time to sit around and chat on land.

Every day I am grateful for our circle of the greatest and most thoughtful friends. So many face this illness alone and lonely. Keep your circle strong; you never know when you may need them.

Counting Blessings

For the last two days he has been following me around pretty closely. Yesterday he followed me into the bathroom. I said I had to go pooh and sent him out to go sit on the couch. When I got out of the bathroom he wasn't on the couch or in the kitchen. I went outside and didn't see him there. I found him in the den, lying on the daybed in the dark.

"Are you tired?" I asked.

"No." he said and got up and proceeded to follow me around.

George is easy to care for so far. He follows directions, he is quiet and loving, he doesn't resist physically or verbally when I direct him. He dresses and bathes himself most of the time. He is even still handling his only medication, eye-drops for glaucoma. I just check. (I really should watch, since sometimes when I ask if he has put them in, he says, "Yes" and then proceeds to go put them in.)

I have many hours of good times with George. George sits on the couch and watches movies or plays Sudoku on his iPad. Some days when I tell him to go sit down, he stays seated and doesn't come follow me around right away again.

When we ride, he is able to ride at regular speed. His tendency to follow me is a blessing then also. We can still go on tricycle adventures together. The other week we rode with friends to Crystal River to see the manatee.

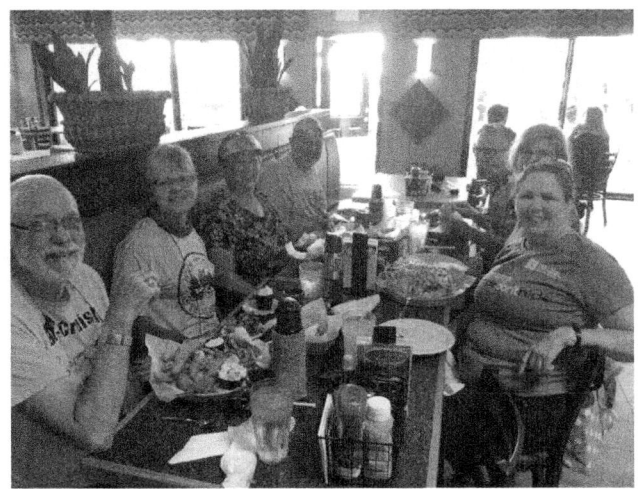

Did I tell you about my Tushy????

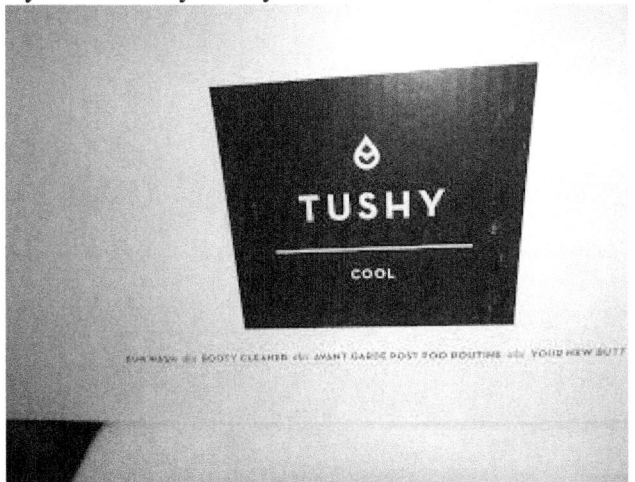

The box says, *"Congratulations! You have seized the bidet! Your butt, the environment and the world will be better off because of it. Install your TUSHY... and flaunt that shiny hiney! Happy pooping."*

It was only $79.

I got it online. I installed it myself. And this morning we got to test it on a very poopy bottom.

Now washing the chunks off is easy. Yeah!!! Every caregiver should have a Tushy!

SUSAN STRALEY

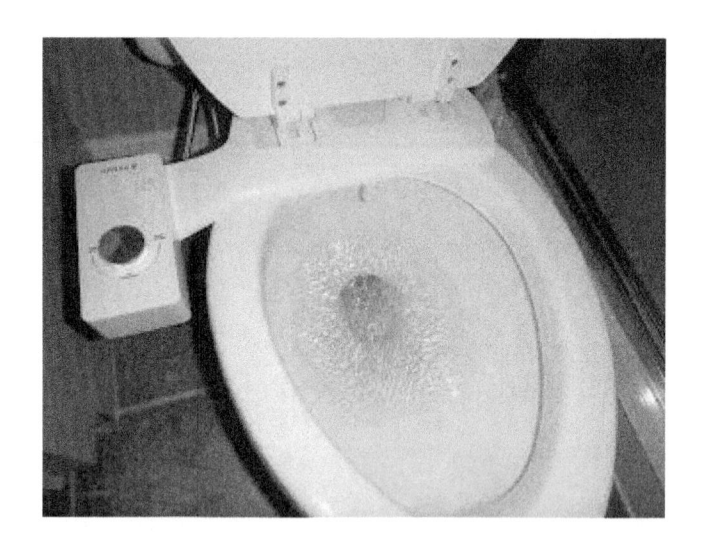

Lucky Enough To Be SAVVY

It is a Sunday and it is too warm to hike or ride bike. The fitness club isn't open very long on Sundays. The pool is so warm already it is no longer refreshing. Florida summer has arrived early. It isn't even May yet.

I decide to clean a bit. I have a guest coming on Monday, and I want to wash windows and freshen up the guest bath and bedroom. But first I have to satisfy George. He is looking at me and following me expectantly. We usually have something to do, and he is anxious to get doing it, whatever it is.

I find a beginner's class of yoga on www.doyogawithme.com. I hooked my iPad up to the big-screen TV, and we spent 40 minutes doing easy yoga and another 15 doing a senior fitness class I found on YouTube. He especially needs to do squats so he can continue to get in and out of his trike. The class has squats, but George doesn't know how to do them, even hanging onto a chair. "Stick your butt out back," I command. "Chest up." I am frustrated. How much do I push? This is important to my longevity as a caregiver. He has to be able to walk and get in and out of chairs and bed.

Once done with the exercises, I set up George with a movie from Amazon Prime. Last night he had watched this TV series for a couple hours, so I was hopeful he would find it interesting this morning. I grab the Windex and my vinegar spray and take one last look at him before I head upstairs. He is looking at me expectantly. "I am going upstairs to clean the bathroom. You stay here. I will be right back."

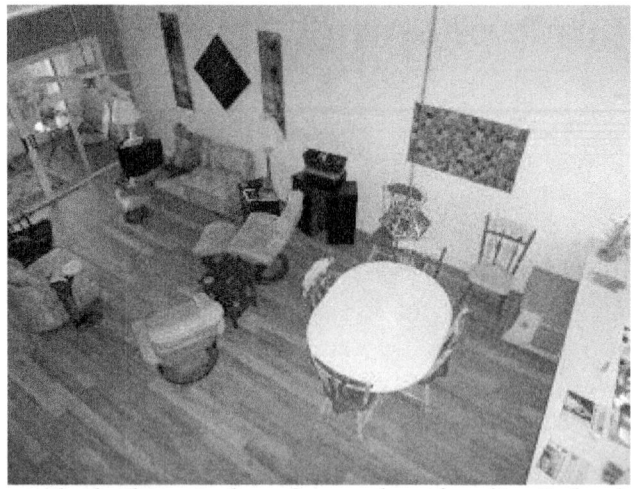

He can see the bathroom door from where he sits. I check on him and he is standing looking up at me. "I am cleaning the bathroom, George. I will be down in a minute. You stay there." He sits back down.

I clean the bathroom and then head into the bedroom and start cleaning the window.

"Sue!" I hear. It is George, already seeking me out.

"I am upstairs!" I yell, and realize that I am facing the window, and the window is open. Now I am sure all the neighbors know that I am upstairs, but George doesn't.

"Sue! Where are you?" he calls out.

I turn around this time and yell away from the window, "UPSTAIRS."

George comes upstairs. I give him my dirty paper towels and tell him to throw them away "downstairs, in the kitchen."

He does. Two minutes pass. "Sue?"

I go to the balcony and tell him that I am right there. I will be done in a little while. I want to do this work myself. I don't need his help, I tell him. I have told him this many times over the years so he is used to me talking to him like that. (Essentially, I don't want your help. Go away now.) This must have satisfied him, because he sat down and I didn't hear from him again. I even got to vacuum the upstairs and then work in the kitchen making chili without his interference.

SAVVY Caregiver Training

The free Savvy Caregiver Training class meets on Wednesday afternoons. I have been taking George to the Key Day Care in Lecanto (about 20 miles away from home) and then finding stuff to do until the caregiving training class starts.

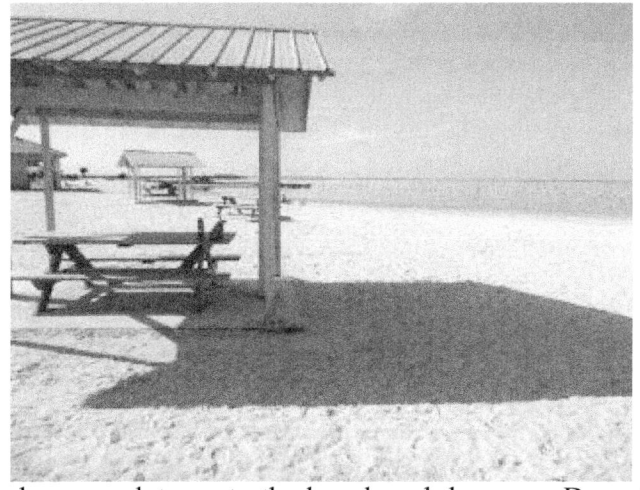

I decided one week to go to the beach and do yoga. Doesn't that sound nice? I got excited about the idea. Each week, drop him off, and go do yoga on the beach.

But I found out there are tiny biting bugs on the beach. A really good Yogi would be able to ignore the tiny bites or just not judge the bites as bad or uncomfortable. But I am not a good Yogi. I could not ignore them and decided that yoga on the beach wasn't such a great idea after all.

There is a bus!

I found out through another wife/caregiver in the SAVVY class about the bus that comes to Inverness. It took me several calls and paperwork, but I finally got the bus coming to our house to pick up George on Wednesdays and Fridays. It takes him to the Key Training Center Adult Day Care. It costs $5 one way. I still pick him up because the last pick up by the bus at the Key Training Center is at 1 p.m. I pick him between 4 and 5 p.m.

George is good with it! I just put him on the bus and off he goes. It is run by the Citrus County Transit. Thank you very much!

In the SAVVY class I have met other wife caregivers. After training I hope to have them gather with me with and without their spouses. It could be kind of a "Demented Wives Club." Some of them are already meeting on Friday evenings with their spouses at a local Veterans Center for dinner and dancing.

Levels and Stages of Dementia

Part of SAVVY Caregiving Training is educating us about the different levels or stages of the illness. For example, the Alzheimer's Association makes it simple with Early Stage, Mid Stage, and Late Stage. Then it is easy for me to say that George is in Mid Stage.

But they also have an Allen measurement. One of our homework assignments was to determine at what Allen level our loved one is. The Allen measurements start with 6 being normal and 1 being bedridden and close to death. We were shown videos of people at the different levels. It was depressing. I sit next to a woman. She is saying, "I don't want to do this!" I rub the back of her shoulders.

As a caregiver, she is fairly new at it. Her husband suddenly showed dramatic symptoms in October and was diagnosed not long after that. She is still struggling with denial and wishing it away. I am grateful to be at the stage I am, with George as easygoing as he is. I am reminding myself, "These are the good old days."

Anyway, level 3 is the level where they are usually put into a memory care unit because they have a hard time understanding instructions and can't do much for themselves.

The next week in SAVVY I told them where I thought George was and why.

4 or 4.5 because he gets up, dresses himself, sometimes even changing his disposable pants and washing himself off. He makes the bed. He prepares his own cereal. At night he remembers his one

medication most of the time. He can sometimes say full sentences that are on topic and make sense.

I also said that he is sometimes a 3. Sometimes I have to get in the shower with him and help him because he just knows to wash from the waist down. He is not aware of the rest of his body. I sometimes have to guide him to get dressed later in the day. Sometimes I have to guide him to his chair. He has both urinary and bowel incontinence. I have to remind him to drink water and hand him the bottle of water.

I am glad to be taking the class.

What Else?

I am still working part-time at Trailside Bike in Floral City.

Working is good, it is distracting, I am still contributing, and I am making a bit of income to help cover extra costs (more shorts for George as he gains weight, more disposable pants).

My sister, Mary, came for a ten-day visit! Since I was picking her up late at the airport I reserved a place for us to spend several nights closer to the east coast of Florida. It was an organic farm. George and I arrived early and checked in before picking up my sister and we enjoyed watching the animals.

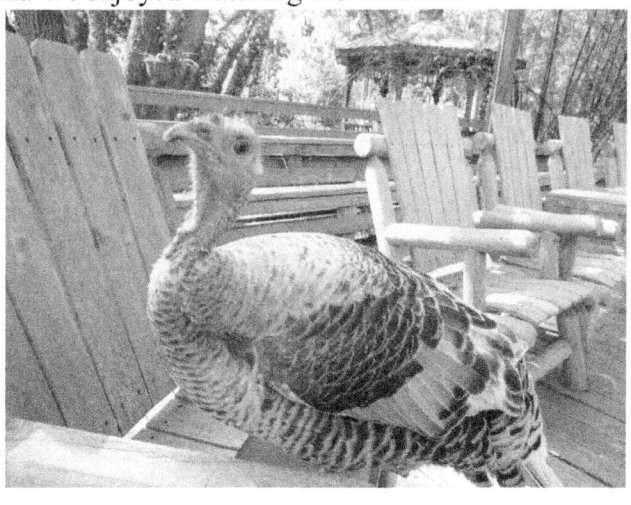

But our lodging was a storage shed with lofts and ladders. The bathrooms were off in a bunkhouse. I got permission from the owner to enter the men's bathroom to help George. It really was a neat place to stay if we were younger and not living with dementia. It wasn't exactly dementia comfortable.

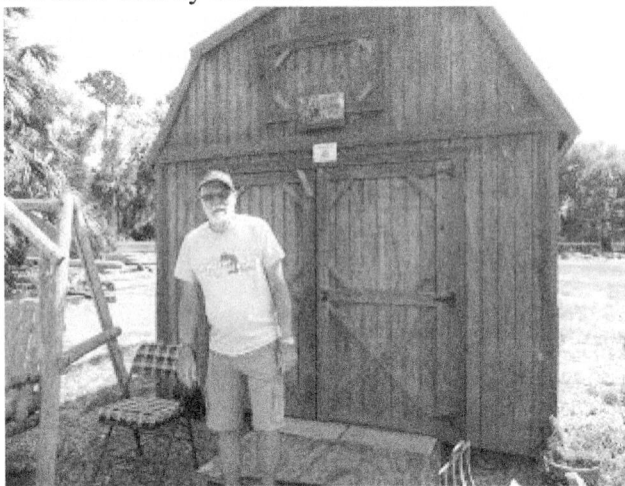

It was super-great seeing my sister again.

On our last trip to the wash-house/bathroom in the evening we almost walked through a huge spider web across our path.

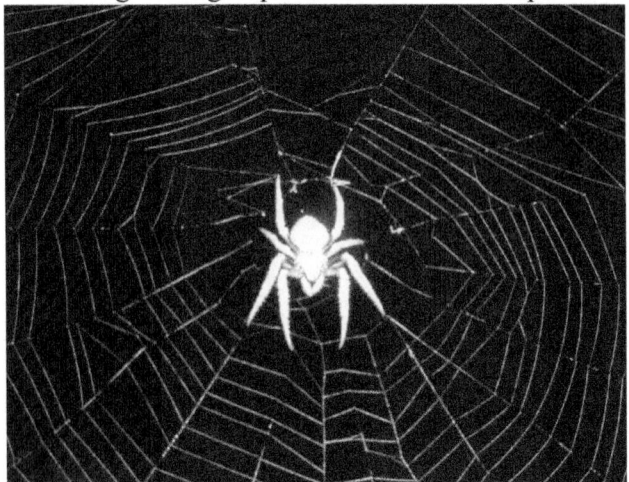

On the way back, we forgot about it and George got really tangled in it. Fortunately, I could see the spider still on a remaining strand high above George's head. It was funny watching George try to get the sticky web off of his arms and hands.

I didn't sleep well. In the early morning, before sunrise, when Mary suggested we just pack up and head home right away, I was in agreement. Thank you to Sunshine Farms for the refund on our additional nights.

Mary's stay was awesome. We were able to walk and talk. One day, George went to day care and Mary and I kayaked on the Rainbow River. It is a crystal clear spring-fed river. And we got the shuttle to the top so we only had to go downstream.

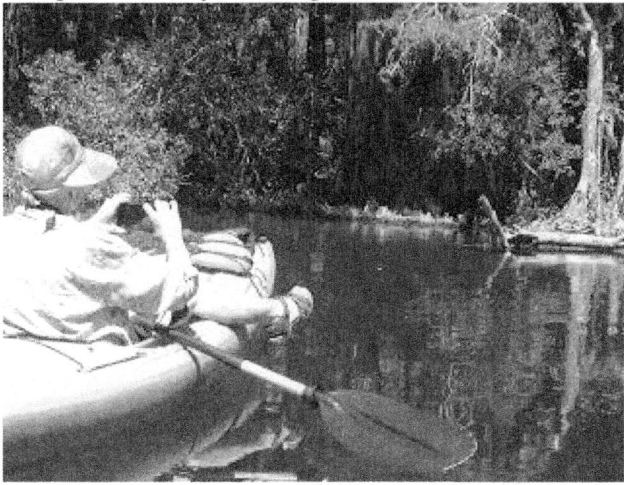

After a week, Mary said to me, "You are doing an awesome job with George."

That meant a lot to me because she herself is a very caring and kind caregiver. She provided care for our mom who had dementia. She also has some clients she helps several times a week.

She saw me in action one day when George was following me around real close like there was a string attached to me and him. I was losing my patience. I kept asking him what he wanted. He would just laugh his nervous laugh and not know or be able to tell me. I tried to set him up with an activity, but he just got up and followed me anyway.

That time, she was able after a while to get him to do some activity with her so I could breathe and get something done.

Another time he was following me like that and he finally told me that he wanted sex. I said, "Well, OK. You go in the master bathroom and take care of that yourself."

He wouldn't do it, but it put an end to that episode of following me around. This is difficult. My life partner and lover... am I wife or nurse-maid? How can I wash his butt and then....

On Friday when I picked him up from the Training Center after I finished work, he had a picture he had made for me. He had told the aide, "Sue will know what it means."

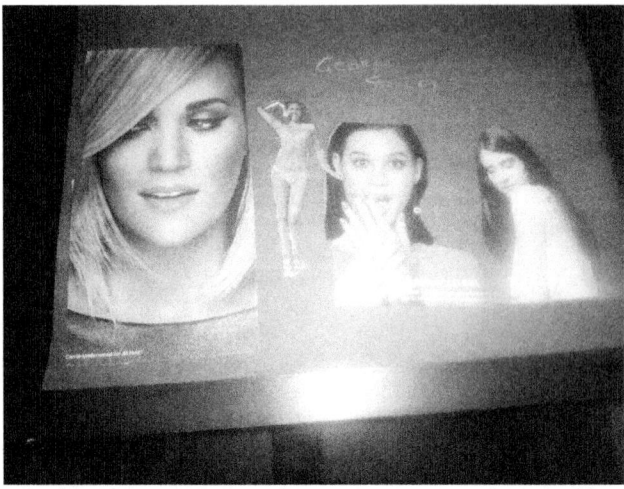

I am sure this is an issue that every caregiver-wife faces. I brought it up in SAVVY class as a topic I wanted to discuss with other wives. I really don't know if I need to discuss it. It is what it is.

My sister returned home, the last of the snowbirds are leaving and life is getting very quiet here. Debra and Glen came over yesterday to test out our snorkel equipment in the community pool.

There is an aqua-aerobics class at the public pool that I have been going to with Debra. I bring George and his coloring book and I wave to him throughout the class. He seems content to just watch and color. It works! Life is good.

Towels and Pre-arrangements

May 8, 2017

Towels

OK, let's talk towels. I catch myself trying to teach, trying to lecture, and trying to control the towel situation. But it is out of my control these days.

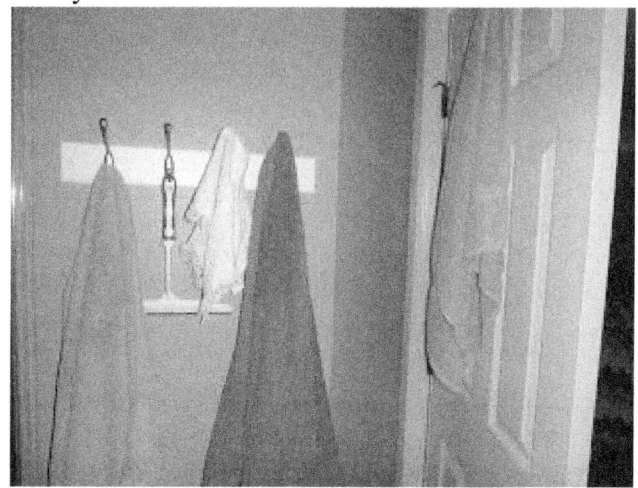

First there were the kitchen towels. George likes to help in the kitchen. Any spot on the counter or in the sink he is attracted to and wants to wipe up. Which is good, right? My kitchen has never looked so spotless.

He helps unload the dishwasher. I hand him a clean dish towel. He dries a dish and puts it away. And while at the cupboard he sees a spot of jam or coffee and wipes it up with his clean towel. He wipes his beard and mustache. Then he comes back to get another dish.

At first I tried to teach him, to train him. But unlike a child, people with memory loss do not learn. Yet we as caregivers are supposed to help them remain involved, and household tasks are a good area to keep them involved.

A friend who also has a husband with dementia was visiting one day. She picked up a towel hanging on the stove handle drying and asked, "Is this for the dishes or for the hands?" I wanted to laugh. My mind shouted, "THERE ARE NO MORE DISTINCTIONS! THE LINES DO NOT EXIST!!!" But I got her a clean towel without saying a word. I picked up the towel on the stove handle and went to the garage and put it on my "dirty-towel/rag line."

My friends Richard and Louise hung some clotheslines in the garage for me this winter. One line is always covered with rags and towels.

But the kitchen isn't the only place where my blood pressure rises over towel issues.

You see, George... sigh.

You need to first know that in the first 39 years of marriage and doing laundry for George I never *ever* saw a brown spot on his underwear or any towel. He was super clean, meticulous, and methodical. I admired that in him, his cleanliness - his attention to the little things. His shower and drying and clipping were reliably the same.

So you can imagine my surprise when I went to grab a towel to dry my face and there was a brown spot.

I have tried different things. I have tried reminding him not to "dig in" with the towel. I have tried wet wipes, but he still wants to dry with a towel after the wet wipes. I have tried hanging *my* towel on the back of the door and letting him know and reminding him that that is *my* towel. I have tried different colors, different places, and monitoring him when he dries himself.

"*No poopy towels*," I say in a joking way. We smile. I know it won't stick. After all, he has progressive dementia. At least he dries himself.

I am learning in SAVVY Caregiver Classes that there will be a time when his skin becomes too sensitive. The shower won't feel good; the towel will seem very rough no matter how soft.

These are the good old days. I am grateful he can still dry himself and dress himself. I talk myself down from the instant emotion of revulsion and anger when I reach for a towel and it is soiled. I have learned to look the towels over for stains. I turn my anger into energy to take the towel to the laundry area and pre-treat it. Then hang it on the rag-line. It is another caregiver adaptation.

Pre-arrangements

It is Wednesday morning, May 3rd. I have arranged for George to take the bus to the Key Training Center. The past two times the bus has picked him up exactly at 9 a.m. I have arranged to meet with someone from the Neptune Society to make pre-paid cremation arrangements for George. She is to arrive at 9:15 a.m. I am feeling proud of myself for arranging the timing of these two items so well.

George and I get some folding chairs and go sit in the shade by the curb waiting for the bus. But 9 a.m. comes and goes and the bus does not arrive. I call the transit office and I learn they are coming at 9:45.

The woman from Neptune Society shows up at 9:15. I bring out another chair for her. She starts going through her presentation. I explain to her that George has dementia and the arrangements are for him. She tells me about her mother with dementia.

She asks George questions and he does OK. But he is crying and wiping away tears. He knows what is going on. Finally the bus comes and George is instantly up and ready to go. He is excited and the session with the Neptune lady is forgotten. Thank goodness for that.

I get him on the bus and pay the driver. When I return to my chair I see that the Neptune lady is crying. She apologizes. I tell her that George and I are still having fun together. This wasn't just about George; she is processing the loss of her mother to the illness.

Pre-arranged funeral/burial is an "ignored" asset. What I mean is it is ignored when and if we have to apply for help from Medicaid. I as the surviving spouse get to keep that asset. Not that it is an asset... it's an expense really.

I buy the package. They charge a bit over $1,000 for the funeral trust and a bit over $1,000 for a "box" that they give you with a booklet for you to fill out with all the stuff your survivors will need in order to settle your affairs after you pass. You can't buy the trust without the box. It is how they get away with keeping 1/2 the cost for their current expenses.

Keeping Active

Sunday morning George and I go for a walk.

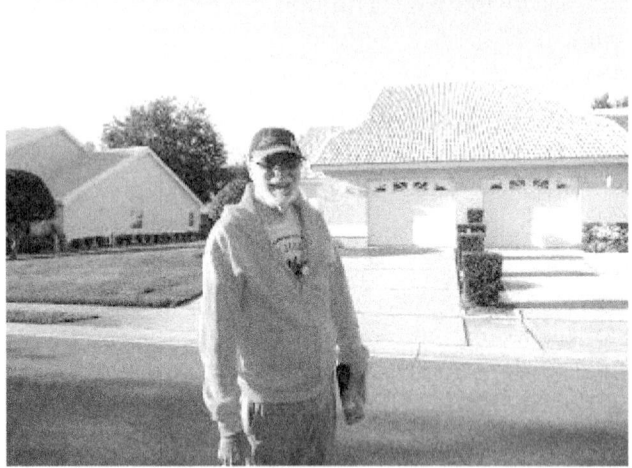

I take us up the trail where we pass the farm animals that the middle school raises. They currently have a fuzzy chicken and a horny turkey.

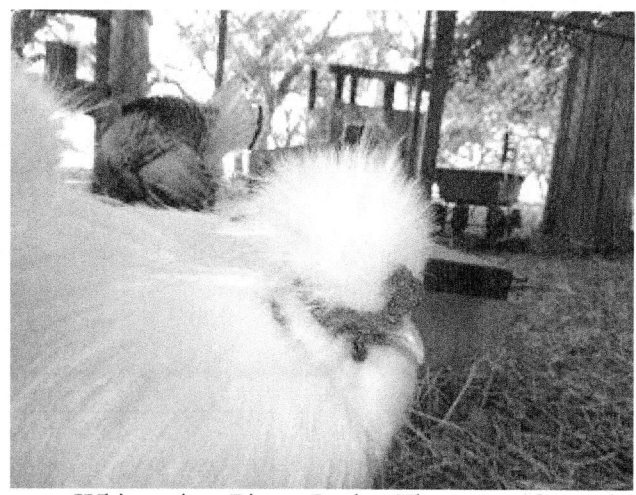

I take us to Whispering Pines Park. The route from the trail is steep and uneven. But George is doing well and manipulates it a little slow and awkward but he gets up the incline OK. We walk about two miles in the park.

By the time we get back to that steep slope, George is leaning to his right and walking pretty slow. I am worried he will stumble down the slope. He manages it and we finally get home. I decide no more physical activity for a while. I need to give him time to recover. After he keeps following me around at home I realize I need to get him settled. I set him down with a beverage and a snack and his iPad.

After lunch we are sitting outside on our patio when I hear a knock on our front door. It is Debra and Glen! They were out riding around and decided to stop by. How wonderful to have such good and casual friends. We visit for a while and start talking about our plans to get to the beach this month. We pull out the iPad, find a place in New Smyrna Beach, and book it while we are sitting there. I am feeling bad about spending the money on the motel. Debra says, "Just do it!"

After they leave I feel the wide open space of the rest of the day and I need to fill it. I can't just... be; especially when I have George standing in front of me looking at me expectantly. It is as if he is saying, "Well that was fun. What's next?"

I have wanted to return to the Van Fleet Trail in the afternoon. I think we might see more wildlife on that trail through the wilderness if we do it later in the day.

I pack up snacks and water and our trikes and I drive us over to the Van Fleet Trail. About 50 minutes of driving for a shorter late afternoon ride.

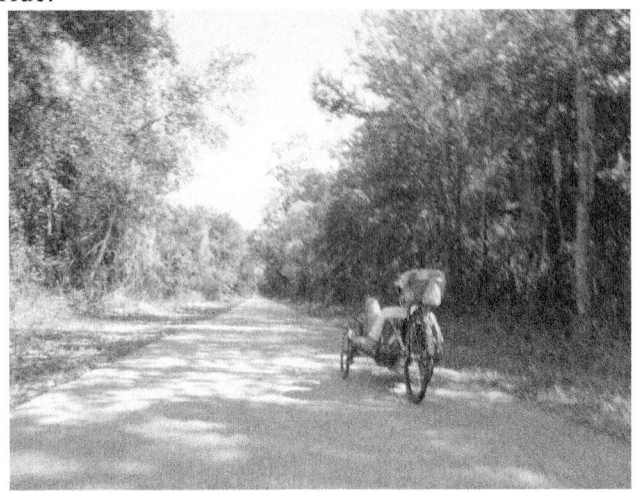

We saw an owl on the ground right next to the trail.

The swamp is very dry. A month ago when we did the trail a pond had two large gators in it. Now the pond is a mud puddle. One gator and her young share the tiny pool of water. WE NEED RAIN!!!

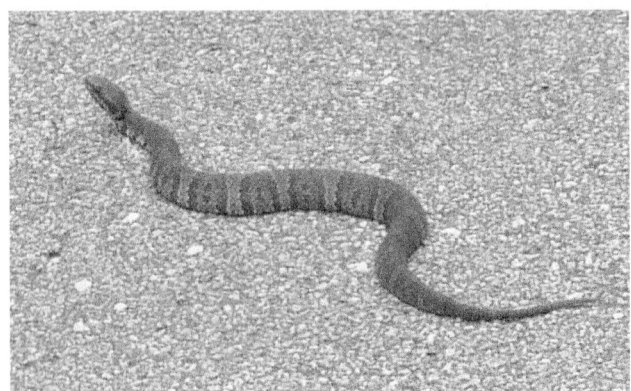

When we were driving into the parking area I saw a large all-white cow lying down near the road and I wondered about her, the way she was laying was strange.... Was she pregnant? On the way out she was standing next to the road licking a black newborn calf that was standing on trembling legs. Its umbilical cord dangled from its belly, still bright red. Yes, she *was* pregnant. But not anymore!

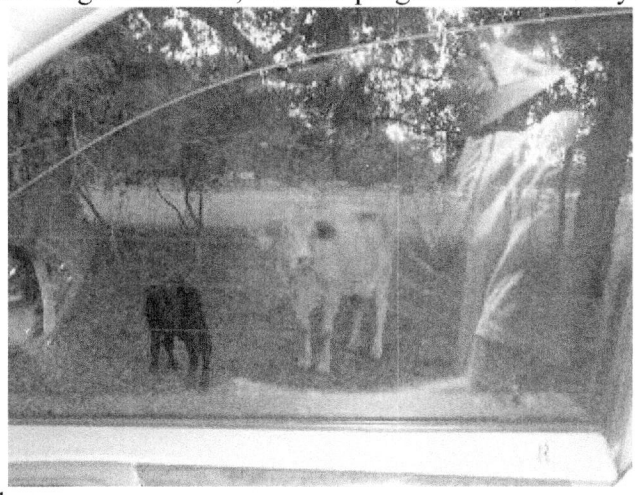

Altogether we saw:
Tortoise
Owl
Sandhill crane
Swallow-tail kite
3 snakes

I asked my boss for the summer off, since business was slow at the bike shop with all the snowbirds flying back home. He said, yes. So I feel now like my time is wide open. It feels uncomfortable to me.

In-Home Respite Care

I got a call from CeCe, a caseworker who interviewed me about getting in-home help. They said I am up on the waiting list and now I could get the in-home help. And at first I refused. I said, "It isn't time yet. George is easy to care for right now." But then I realized I was paying $60 a week for an extra day at the Day Care when all I needed was a few hours to myself. So I called her back and said yes. She came and interviewed. George remembered his social security number, our address and more. Figures he would perform well when they are checking his need for assistance.

She said help will be calling me in about two or three weeks to schedule. I get two days a week for three hours. It will cost me about $125 a month. Thank you, Citrus County and Medicaid or Medicare!

Shadowing

I learned in the SAVVY Caregiver class that there are several behaviors that dementia patients have as a coping mechanism for confusion and fear of what is happening. Some strike out, some are mean, and some, like George, shadow. So he follows me around when he is unsure. This is good to know. Now I am aware that I need to stop what I am doing and get him otherwise occupied and assure him he is OK. That will keep my shadow as happy and content as possible.

Feels Like a Speeding Train

May 11, 2017

Not quite like a speeding train, but sometimes it feels like it....
It is going too fast!
It has been two years since George's definitive diagnosis of chronic progressive dementia "most likely becoming Alzheimer's Disease." I now feel it is moving too fast.

I have heard from others that a person can stay at the same capacity for a long time and then take a step down in what they are capable of and stay there for a while. It seems to me that George took a step down earlier this spring and now it seems he has "stepped down" again.

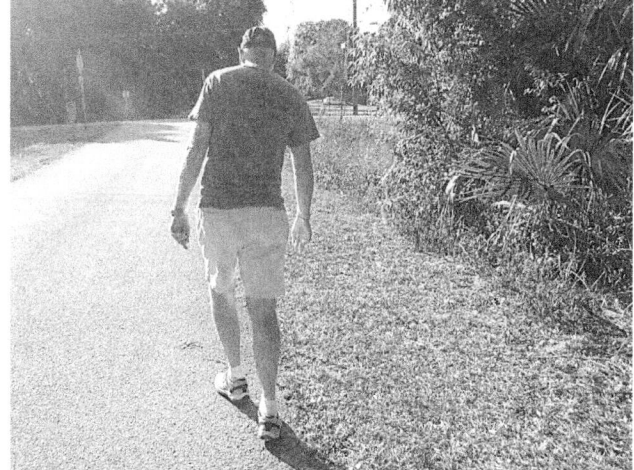

A one-mile walk can start him leaning right and it seems like it is real hard work for him to finish the walk. The exercises we do, elbow to opposite knee, can seem impossible for him to do.

I kind of feel guilty about using movies as a George-sitter. This is silly. He has always loved to sit and watch movies and TV shows. We gave up having a TV in the 90's. But whenever he got a chance... such as in a motel room or when the internet got good enough to stream videos, he'd spend hours and hours watching. I called it wasting his life away. He didn't see it that way.

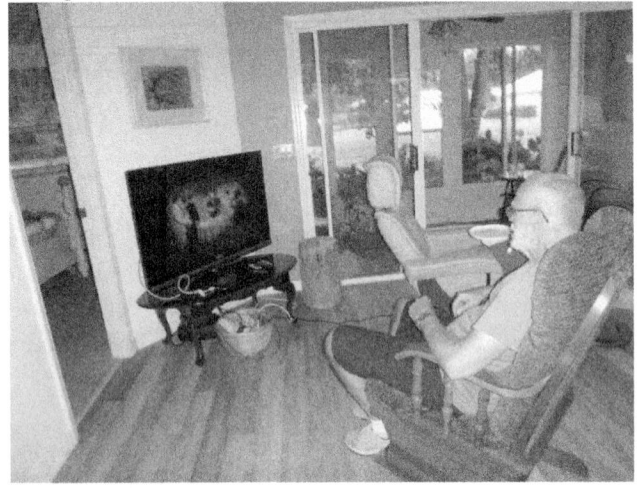

Symptoms of Decline

When I get the yoga mat out to do yoga he follows along in his own way. I no longer try to stand over him and correct him. When we get down on the floor, he lays down with his head up on the seat of the chair. I tell him to scoot down so his head can get on the ground. But he can't figure out how. He doesn't know the technique or he is too weak. I don't know which. I pull on his legs to slide him down, but the yoga mat is doing its job and not sliding on the floor or allowing his bottom to slide down the mat.

OK. I move the chair. He lies there, holding his head up off the floor. I have to instruct him to let his head down. I try to complete my yoga ignoring him and paying attention to my own body. This is an extra yogi challenge. I still benefit from the session but I wonder if George is injuring himself. The next morning he gets up and complains of being stiff. He has a hard time standing up from a sitting position.

We usually bike 32-40 miles on Thursdays. But George was weak today. While we were biking he was lagging farther behind than normal. When we stopped at a restroom I had to help him unclip his shoes from the pedals. I checked his tires and brakes.

I had to help him out of his trike every time we stopped. We biked 17-18 miles. He was definitely ready to quit. I was thinking this wouldn't happen for a long time... this riding shorter and slower. Actually, I wasn't thinking about it much at all, because he was riding so well. I was thinking it would be one of the last things to go.

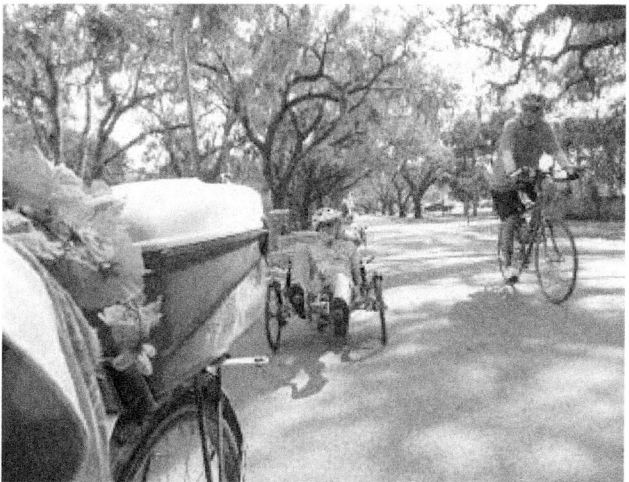

Is this a fluke? Is he just sore and weak this week? How much longer will we have the ability to bike together? If I can't bike I will go nuts. I will be using my respite time to bike with friends. And that is sad because as long as he bikes I know that that part of him is still there. My riding partner is rolling with me.

This is progressing too fast!

We have a date to go over to Debra and Glen's for dinner tonight. It will be good to laugh and be with good friends especially since we missed dining with our bike group today. Life is still very, very good.

Respite Care Adjustments

Yesterday, at 9 a.m., I got the folding chairs out and set them on the front sidewalk in the shade. We waited for the bus for an hour. Our neighbor, Pat, was outside and asked George if he was going off to work. George nodded. The bus company gives me an hour window for pick up. So at the end of the hour I called them. It turned out George wasn't on the schedule for being picked up today!

It was on my calendar. How come it wasn't on theirs? I feel a little less competent, a little less organized. We roll with it, get in the car and I drive him to the Key Training Center. He is happy to be there. They are playing corn-hole (bean bag toss) when we arrive. He joins in right away.

I go off to shop and attend the SAVVY Caregiver training. Just before class starts I get a call from our caseworker. She said the grant money at the end of the fiscal year has run out and George will no longer be able to go to the Key Center for free one day a week. He will be able to start up again after July 1st.

The caseworker *also* told me that the in-home care will start in the next couple weeks. They have contacted the provider "Family Life" and they will be contacting me to schedule 12 hours a week until July and then 8 hours a week. She wanted to know how I wanted the hours divided. I said 4 hours, Monday, Wednesday, and Friday.

After thinking about it a while, I wonder if it would be better to get one 6 or 8 hour day. That way I could go kayaking or snorkeling. Is it better to get a few days to do everyday things like go to the gym and shop? We will see.

This in-home care will be subsidized or grant-assisted so that it will cost me less than $200 a month for the help. They will do a bit of house cleaning and put George through some exercises and activities that I give them.

Getting Organized

In SAVVY Caregiver training they talked about being very organized and prepared. Prepared when someone asks "How can I help," with a duty and instructions. Prepared for doctor visits with the medical history, questions, symptoms and observations, list of medications, dosages, prescribing doctor and why prescribed. Arghh!!! Instead of blogging I should be getting organized!

    They talked about doctor visits and I was wondering if I should talk to his doctor already about putting George on palliative care. No treatments unless it makes him more comfortable now. That's the plan, man. Keep him content.

Enjoying Our Moments

June 3, 2017

The Moth is a podcast that I listen to while biking. It is a program that features people telling true stories from their life. I love *The Moth*. It makes me laugh and choke up with tears.

The motto at *The Moth* goes something like this: "You either have a good time or you have a good story." I like that... and I like to think that George and I might be breaking the rules. Maybe we are having fun *and* making a good story at the same time.

I mean, a story can just be about a moment in your life... like one story on *The Moth* today of an eight year old who got up on stage for her school talent show and instead of singing she just stood there and cried she was so scared and so unprepared... for two minutes... with background music, she stopped a moment to gather courage and started to sing and ended up sobbing some more.

I enjoy the stories I hear from my fellow Dementia Divas I met while in SAVVY Caregivers class. Here's one:

"The other thing that my father did today, I had to go the bank and just as I was coming into the house I heard him in the hallway making a lot of noise so I went over to see what he is doing and found him taking the toilet chair out of the bathroom (I had put it in there after he had that fall so he couldn't slip off the toilet again, hopefully). I told him that it is supposed to be in there so that he wouldn't fall off again.

Then he went into his bedroom and parked his walker and proceeded to come out to the living room without it and I told him that he needed it to get around. He threw up his hands and went back to get it. Then he went back to the bathroom and then came out without his walker again and I asked him, "Where is your walker?" And he said in the bathroom where it should be. I again told him that he was supposed to keep it with him wherever he goes so I went into the bathroom and found it on top of the toilet chair and somehow he had got it stuck."

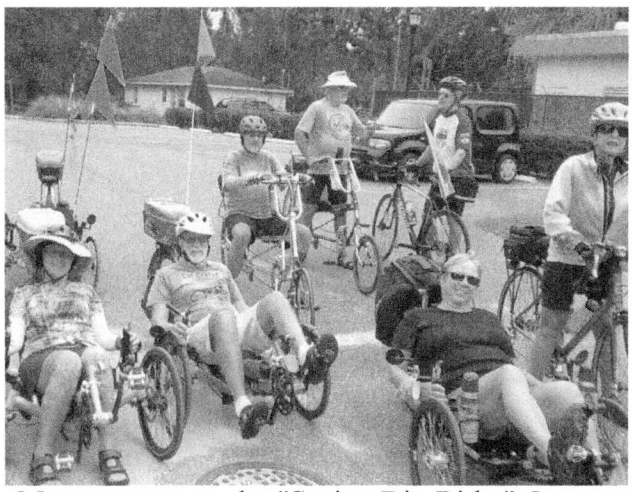

In early May we went on the "Spring Dip Ride." It was a bicycle ride with our bike group that rides a trail and visits three springs starting at Fanning Springs State Park in Fanning Springs, Florida. There were only five riders, but we had a really good time.

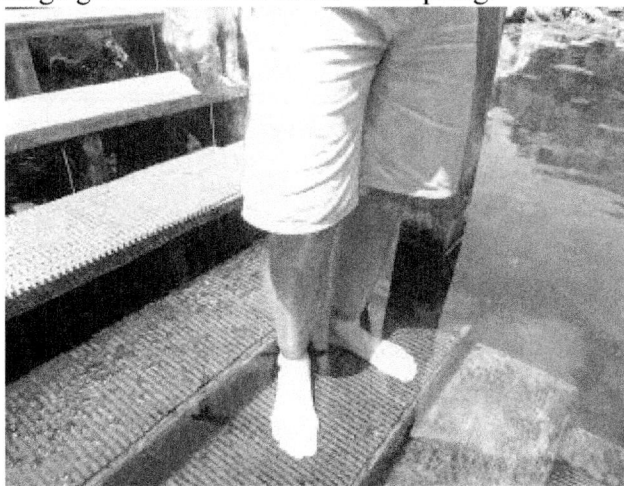

Even George got his feet wet in the first spring.

As you can tell, he rarely takes his socks off. His feet are very white... like Socks the cat.

We continue to ride as often as we can with our bike group.

Respite Care Rescue

I now have in-home help that comes and provides "respite care" twice a week. The agency sent me a caregiver. The only time this caregiver is available is on our group ride days. She can only do four hours at a time, she says. I am happy to have some time when I don't have to keep one ear listening for George.

I have her come at 2:30 so we can ride our trikes and shower beforehand.

I graduated from the SAVVY Caregiver class and treated myself to a full day with George at the Key Training Center.

I met up with Glen and Debra and went on a test snorkel swim in the Rainbow River. The Rainbow is a clear spring-fed river about half an hour from our home.

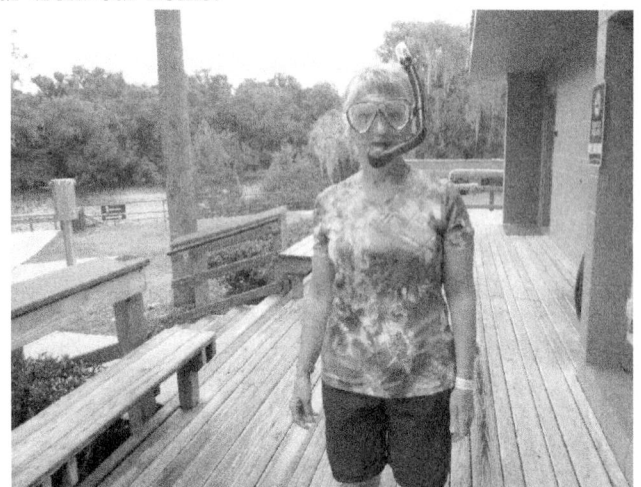

Sometimes figuring out what to do with my four hours of respite is perplexing. It is too hot to go for a fast walk. Sometimes I am too tired by that time of day to go to the gym. Sometimes I shop, once I got my hair cut, and often I spend the time reading or catching up on emails at Panera Bread.

Traveling With Dementia

Our granddaughter turns 15 in June. I really debated about going to visit. It would mean traveling to Wisconsin. My old way of planning is, if we take the time to get there, we should stay a while. But now, being away from home might be hard on George. If it is hard on George, it will be stressful for me.

I booked the flight with a return after only three nights. We will get to see our son and daughter and their families. I will get to see my sister who has arranged for us to meet up with my aunt. It will be a fun-filled few days.

I was worried about not being able to sit with George on the plane. That would make it more stressful for him. I reserved our seats together on the way... pre-seat assignment charges apply.

We are going with just a few clothes that will rinse out and I will buy a package of Depends when we arrive. Only one 8 x 14 x 18 bag allowed per person free of charge. It will work. Another adventure....

Margarita Surprise

George hasn't drunk alcohol since sometime in the late 70's. It isn't like he had a problem with alcohol; he just decided one day that he was tired of feeling crappy the next day after drinking so he just stopped. No crossing the line with a drink or even a taste of mine.

Friday night this week we went for Mexican food in The Villages with Debra and Glen. I ordered a small margarita and it turned out is was BOGO night. (That is two for the price of one.) The waiter delivered two margaritas to the table at once. Neither Debra nor Glen wanted my second margarita. So there it was sitting on the table by me and George. George took a sip. Debra and I looked at each other, our eyes as wide as saucers. We didn't say anything. George drank the whole glass.

Lots of fun times. We ain't done yet!

We Are The Fortunate Ones!

June 16, 2017

If uncontrollable pooh is your biggest problem, you are blessed.

Those are my words of wisdom for today.
Nature greets us right outside our front door.

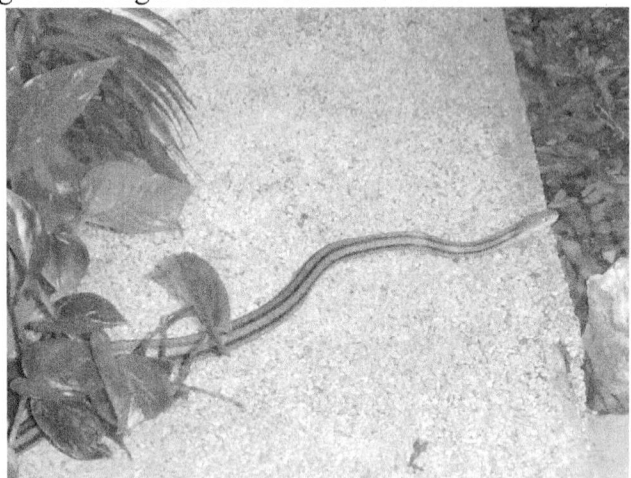

Friends, family and the community at large continue to step in to support us again and again.

Flight to Wisconsin

Our trip to Waukesha went wonderfully. George must have understood that I needed time to myself to pack. He agreed to watch a movie and I packed our bags. Just two personal bags allowed for free on Frontier. I packed four Depends and two washrags in baggies just in case.

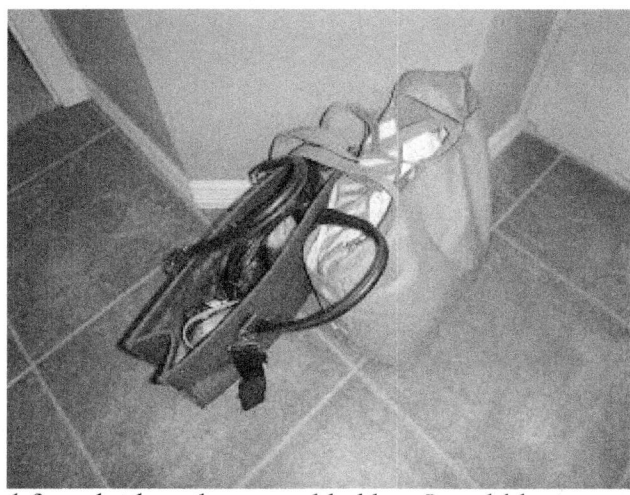

I figured for a lot less than an added bag I could buy a small package of Depends once we arrived in Wisconsin.

George was a little nervous waiting for the flight and on the plane. He gave a nervous giggle each time there was an announcement on the sound system. I put in his earbuds and turned on the music on his iPod and he visibly seemed calmer and the nervous giggles stopped immediately. Like magic! Thank you, Apple. A couple times I told him to watch the bags while I went into the bathroom or to get us a cup of coffee. He stayed put.

There is a great documentary on the magic of music in Alzheimer's patients. If you are a caregiver, a good thing to have is an iPod with your loved one's favorite songs on it.

Our son Jeremy and his family had us over for dinner on the night we arrived. My granddaughter gave George and me wonderful "hello" hugs.

So many to thank; I will send a personal email to each. I can't believe it, but each time we dined out someone was paying for our meal! All I can say is, all those good friends and family who send us good thoughts and prayers... THEY ARE WORKING! Keep it up. And to those who contributed and participated in our wonderful trip, *thank you*.

George's daughter Jodie and son-in-law surprised us with an early arrival at the motel where they stayed with us two nights. Jodie arrived in time to dance with her dad at the downtown Waukesha street party.

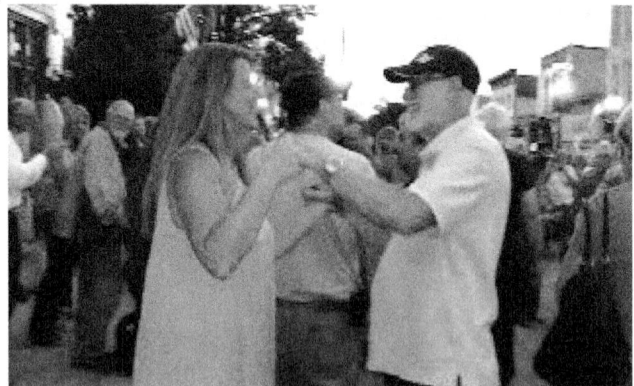

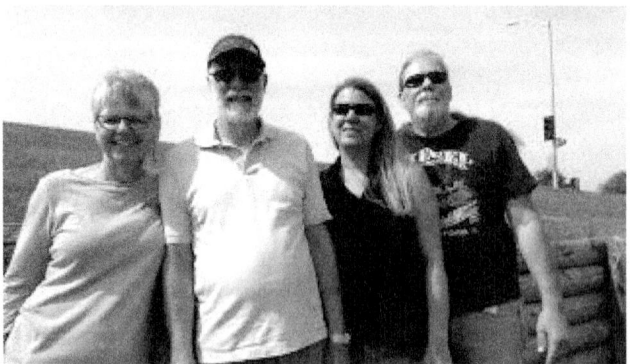

My sister and brother-in-law also drove many hours to spend a couple days with us.

Since they all were at the same motel as us, I could say, "Keep an eye on George, I have to run up to the room..."

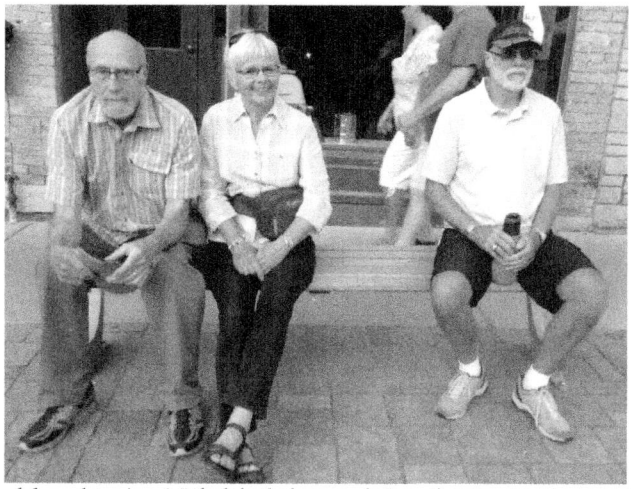

My granddaughter's 15th birthday celebration was at a park on a very windy day. We had to hang onto our potato chips and salad or they would have blown right off our plates.

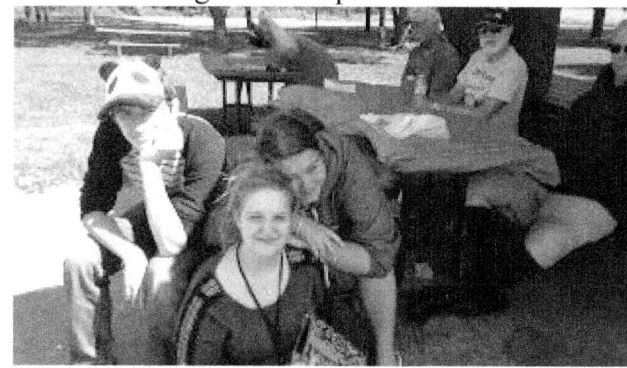

Scent Kit

While we were up north I kept getting alerts on my phone and in my email. An Inverness woman with memory issues went missing. They used the smell dogs and copters and lots of people on the ground searching. It has been a week. There is still no sign of her. The not-knowing what happened must be very hard on her family.

She had wandered before and yet she was still living alone.

I went for a massage on Tuesday upon our return. The masseuse asked me if I had the scent kit for George. "I do!" I said, but then I learned that I did it wrong. I guess I can't touch the pad; it should only have the smell of George on the pad. That is why they don't just use a piece of clothing. There are detergents and other people's smell on clothes.

I will pick up a new scent kit at my next support group meeting.

Preparing the Heart and Mind

So many of us lose ones we love. I have a couple of friends who are currently dealing with having children with terminal illnesses.

I met with a friend who became a widow last June. We talked about how she is working to shape her life and becoming involved in activities and clubs

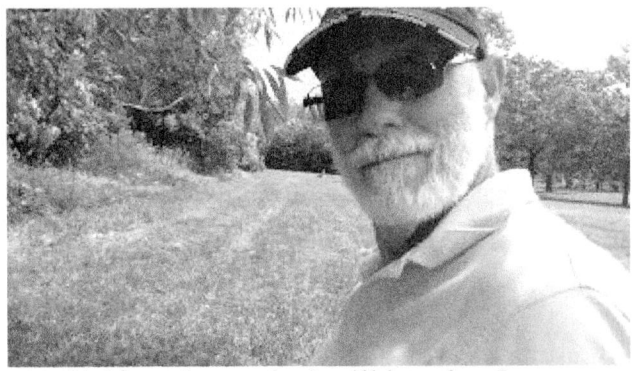

It got me to thinking about who I will be when I am on my own.

Before George started to shadow me and before I got sucked into becoming president of our business, I was involved at times in causes that were dear to me... the environment, justice, equality....

Debra and I were talking the other day and she said what I kind of thought. She said that I was kind of already a widow now. Not really, maybe I am 1/2 a widow. Or maybe 1/3 of me is widow and the other 2/3's of me is able to hug someone, have someone to return to when I am out, have someone to cook for and plan activities for.

Though the silence and lack of conversation are deafening at times, I am far from alone.

I see the respite time I get as being an opportunity to explore who I will become on my own.

Speaking of respite, I got a call from our caseworker. She said a grant opened up again at the Key Training Center. So starting this week George can go back there for two full days a week to the end of June! He and I are both happy about that.

So much joy we still experience daily.

Life in Snippets

"I Have Dementia"

George has been telling people, "I have dementia." Today at breakfast with our bike group, George announced to the group, "I have dementia." And they said, "You are doing very well with it."

Later we were riding our trikes back from the restaurant and a biker (Bill) pulled up next to George and asked how he was doing. George told him, "I have dementia." Bill asked how he was doing with that: "Does it make you sad?"

George said, "No."

Good answer!

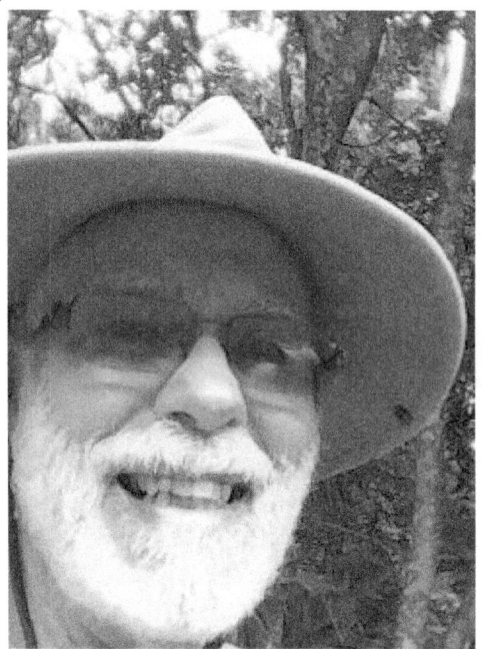

We are walking a loop that goes over two miles. We are toward the end of the walk and George has not slowed down much. As we walk down the street two young and vigorous lawn maintenance workers stop to let us by before crossing the street. George says,

"Hi, how ya doin'?" and they say, "Good, how are you doing?" And George says without missing a beat... "I got dementia."

Friends we see every week will ask George how he is doing and he tells them, "I got dementia." They often look at me not knowing how to reply to that.

"He is living very well with dementia, aren't you, George?" I say. He smiles and does his half crying nervous laugh.

Since George doesn't talk much, I have no idea of how much he is aware. This loop, "I have dementia," may be why he cooperates when I tell him to do things.

Preparing for What's Ahead

The woman with dementia in Inverness who went missing while we were in Waukesha is still missing. I got a new scent kit at a support group meeting, and this time I read the directions. I had George be the only one to touch the gauze and to wipe it on his armpit area only. Then I had him place it in the jar.

Now I have two scent kit jars on the fridge and some pictures of George I had printed at Walgreens.

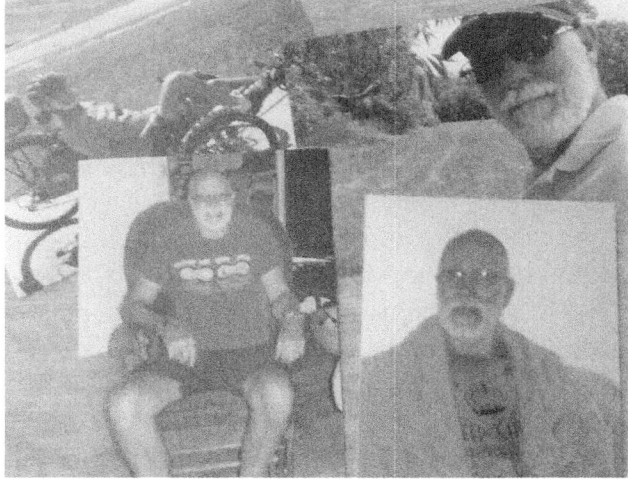

The folks in our support group are frustrated that this is the best they can do on a limited budget. "We put chips in our animals, why can't we chip our people?" they ask.

We talk about available GPS trackers. There is a monthly fee. Getting your person to carry a phone is not reliable.

My next step is to get some *Do Not Resuscitate* forms completed and put on the fridge. And either some extra locks for the doors (that he can't easily see or unlock) or some alarms or bells for the doors.

George doesn't wander now. I sleep in a separate room now, and I don't worry much about him wandering at night.

I know that he gets up at night. He has stayed in the bedroom and attached bath. I know he gets up because sometimes I find two pair of clean disposable underwear in the waste basket. He gets up at night and changes his underwear. He can't tell when they are wet even when he pulls them down and looks. Maybe he is being extra cautious.

I mentioned it to him once, when it first happened. Now... it just is what it is. I fish them out, fold them up, and put them back in the basket with the others.

One night last week he must have soaked the sheets; the tell-tale ring was there. Thank goodness I thought ahead and put on a mattress protector a few months back.

During the day, I ask him if I can check to see if his underwear is wet. He sometimes doesn't comprehend or can't understand why I would be asking him this. So I say, "Pull down your pants." He grins.

It is so much easier to be the caretaker of a spouse. I imagine it would be harder with a parent or sibling in these matters.

Now I shower with him to make sure that he washes his head and armpits, because what he sees (the lower half of his front body) is what he washes. Sometimes he can wash other parts of his body with prompting, sometimes I do it for him, and I smile and tell him how lucky he is to have his favorite lady wash him all over.

For now, once he leaves the shower, I can still stay in the shower. I realize this is a temporary stage. Right now he is able to dry off his body and dress himself. He even thinks to trim his nails sometimes. If he is especially foggy, I lay out his change of clothes for him on the bed.

Words Are Lost

He is losing more and more of his language ability. This morning I told him that he was going to the Key Center. I told him he would be taking the bus. He goes out into the garage and opens the garage door and starts to get the bikes out. I go outside and I say, "No, we aren't taking the bikes today. You are getting on the bus."

He starts again to pull out the trikes. "The bus, George, the bus, not bikes." He looks at me *un*-comprehending. "Bus," I repeat several times. Then I pull out the folding chairs we sit in while we wait for the bus. That is when he gets it. He stops trying to put the bikes out and goes and sits on the chair at the curb.

Bus and Help

When the bus picks up George, I can leave right away and go do something, or I can stay home and just be home without one ear listening. Until I became a caretaker, I had no idea what it was like to constantly have my ear listening for what my person was doing. It is just wonderful to spend a few moments on the toilet or in the garden not having to be ready to jump into action. Thank you, Citrus County, Elder Affairs, and the Key Training Center for respite care.

Sometimes Capacities Are Unknown

I totally underestimated what he could do. I got some 24 piece puzzles and he seemed to be OK with doing them. Then a neighbor brought over some 300 and 500-piece jigsaw puzzles. I am amazed at how he can still do them. It is wonderful because it keeps his attention for hours. Thank you!

The other day he surprised me by asking me, "Do you have Jodie's number?"

"Yes," I said, "do you want me to call her for you?"

He nodded and he talked to her without much prompting on my end. "I got dementia," he told her with his teary giggle.

After he called Jodie, he asked me to call his estranged son. I called and got an answering machine. I prompted George to leave a message. The message machine cut George off too quick. I tried to add, but it also cut me off.

Life Still Interrupts

I dropped my cell phone in the toilet and had to get a new one and set it up. I am glad to have some respite time to take care of this.

I could be working now. I could be building my Social Security pot and retirement accounts. But if I am working, who would take care of George?

My sister advises, "Don't worry, be happy, it will all be good." And yes, I remind myself not to worry about tomorrow. I vow to enjoy today and the moments we have.

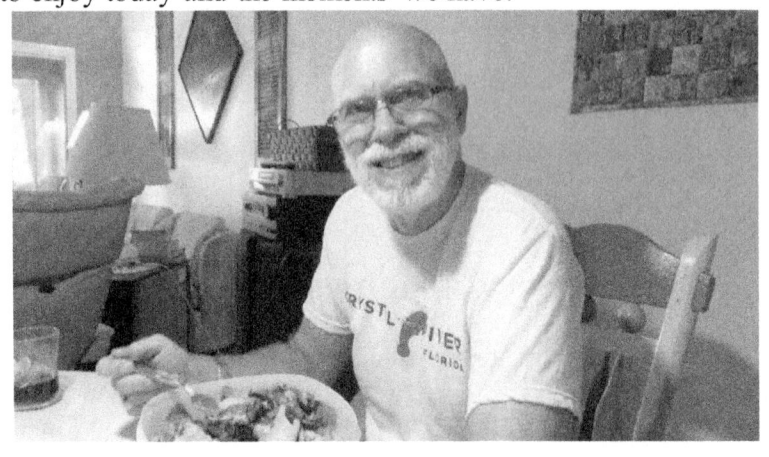

"Will You PLEASE Just Sit and Stay Already?"

July 28, 2017

    George is used to me arranging our lives. Most mornings we go do something. We either bike or walk or go exercise or go *do* something. So after he finishes his breakfast, he is up and ready to go. Sometimes I want to just sit and enjoy my breakfast, drink my coffee, read the paper, check my email.

    BUT NOOOOOO... because he is pulling the bikes out of the garage, or going and standing by the car, or standing at my side waiting, hovering, waiting. I have tried telling him we don't have anything planned right away. I have tried setting him down to do something like color or work a puzzle or watch a movie. But something in him tells him we've got to go do something and he can't stay with the activity. Two minutes, then he is up at my side or out by the car, or pulling out the trikes, or sitting on the curb waiting for the bus.

    I am grateful he likes to go do things. I have women in our support group with spouses who refuse to go anywhere. They won't go to Day Care. We have so much to be grateful for.

    Even with so many losses in George's cognitive ability I still feel such love for him. That is a good thing. It gives me patience and kindness when he is hovering too close for too long.

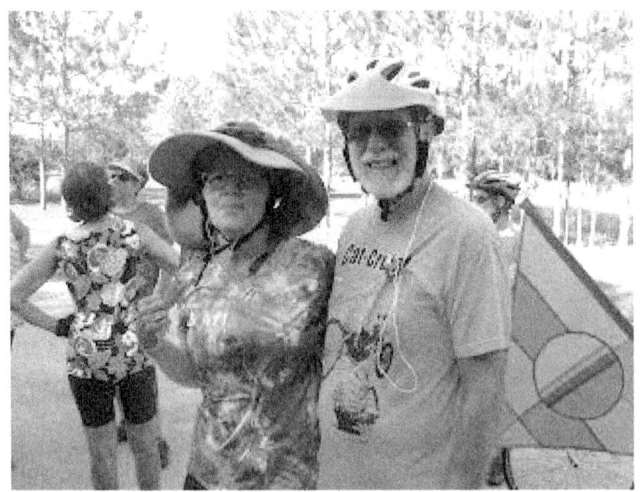

This journey is not without lessons.

Caregiver Pointers

I have mostly learned:

- It is easier to always go *do* something in the morning. Then if I want to relax over the paper, I wait until we return after our activity. Then he can settle in and work on his puzzle or color or watch a movie.
- To store *my* towel hidden from view, hanging on a hook behind the bathroom door. I have also learned to check the towel for poopy spots *before* I dive my face into the towel.
- That smiling at him while I wash him helps him be OK with me taking over this task.
- When he hovers more than usual he might be hungry, or need to go to the bathroom or be cleaned up, or given a hug and reminded we aren't going anywhere and I don't need his help right now.
- If he is shadowing me, I need to stop what I am doing and see if I can get him interested in a task. I need to take care of him first.

- Sometimes he shadows because he wants sex. It is OK for me to say "No."
- To make sure the food is cooled off enough to eat before I put it on the table. Because he just can NOT wait to put big scoops of food in his mouth.
- To touch his arm or distract him when I catch him staring too much and too long at strangers.
- To keep a supply of plastic bags in the bathroom and extras in the bottom of the waste can for easy access.
- That we are very fortunate that he can still walk a distance, bike with me and the group and enjoy dining with others even though he can't talk much or follow the conversation.
- To accept help when it is offered.
- To trust my nose: when I smell pooh it is probably pooh.

I'd like to say that I have learned to enjoy today without worrying about tomorrow. But "learned" means I have arrived fully on the other side of worry.

Maybe it is better to say I am trying... I am striving to put worry into action toward knowledge or a solution and to enjoy our moments and the nature that surrounds us.

The Withlacoochee Bike Trail takes us out into the forest and past ranches and farms. We see hawks and wild turkey and deer and armadillo.

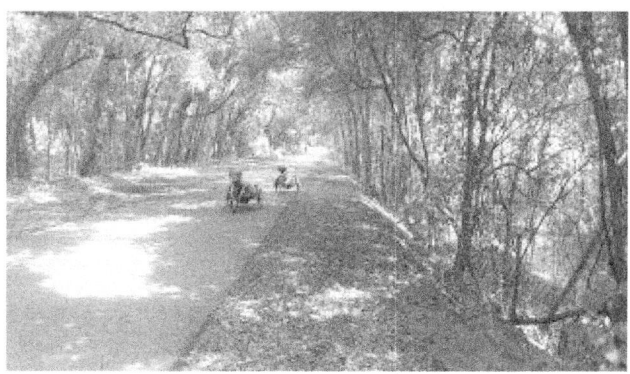

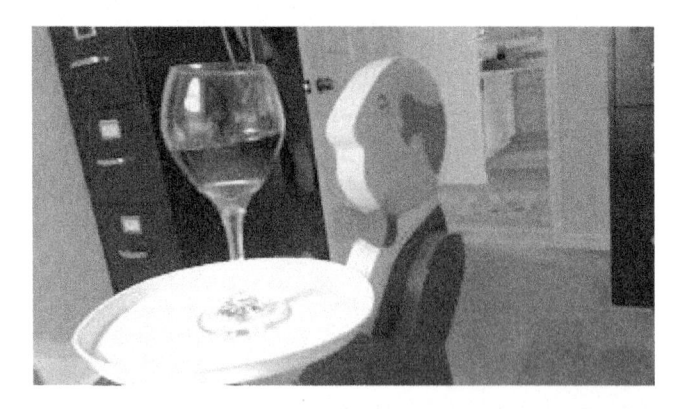

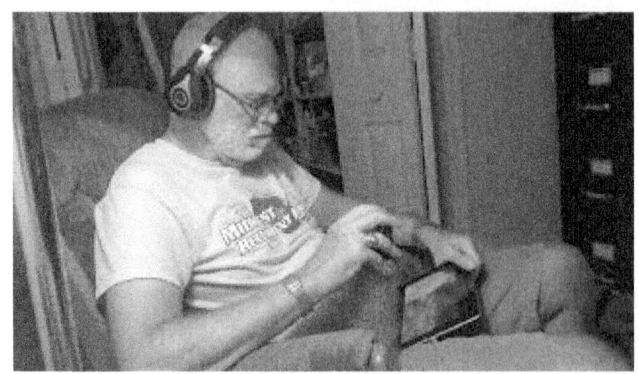

I set George up with a movie and his earphones. After only a minute or two he took them off. I asked him what was wrong. He could not answer. So I turned the volume up a bit and tried again. After another few minutes he took them off again. I asked again. I asked different ways so all he would have to do is nod. He just looked at me, distressed a bit. I tried again. He stuck with it.

I wondered, maybe he needed to go to the bathroom or to move around or to tell me something but he couldn't.

It wasn't until today as I was thinking back that I realized that if he can't understand me and if he can't follow conversations, then movies with lots of dialog are probably not enjoyable anymore. My friend Debra suggested some nature programs with lots of images and music instead of dialog. I will try those next.

At breakfast with our biking friends he told our friend Glen that he has dementia. "How is that working for you?" Glen asked. "Are you doing OK with it?" George nodded and smiled.

I picked up a DNR from George's doctor. This is a doctor's order to not perform CPR or lifesaving efforts if there is no pulse or breathing. I will make copies (they have to be on yellow paper) and place them with George, on his trike, in the car, on the fridge and with the caregivers. He already has "DNR" on his ID bracelet.

I had a dream. George was bitten by a venomous snake and I felt I needed to decide whether to google how the death would progress from the bite before I could decide whether to call 911. This dream must have been triggered by the DNR process.

I have a job interview coming up. Today I ran the numbers. If I have to pay $60 per day for George's care, I will only make about nine dollars a day after taxes working a six-hour day. That is if they pay me more than they would normally pay an Administrative Assistant in Citrus County. It doesn't seem worth it. I would have a net loss.

I am seeking a good clean person to pay to stay in one of our furnished guest rooms upstairs for some extra income. I have to require a minimum stay of three months due to our Home Owner Association's (HOA) regulations.

Stop worrying and go with the flow. It will all work out, says my sister. "It is only money."

Tonight I plan to take George to the VFW for fish and dancing. Flowing, smiling, flowing....

Riding the Waves of Dementia and Caregiving

August 12, 2017

George and I have a good life. We enjoy friends and nature almost every day.

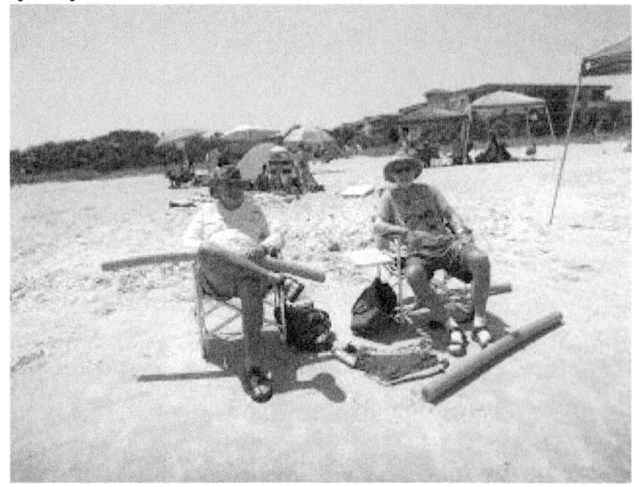

We enjoy food and music.

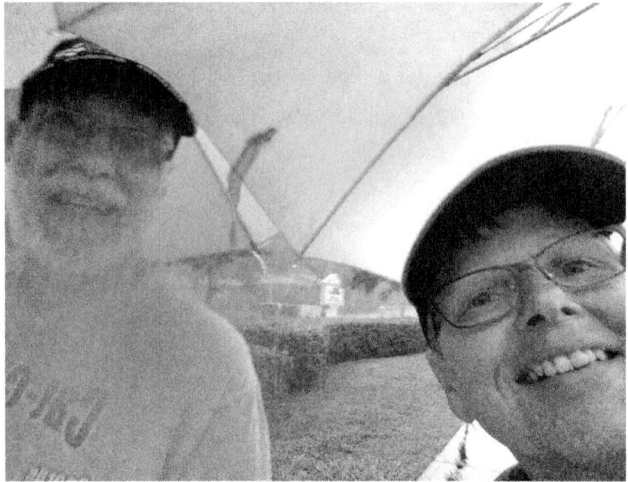

We get movement every day several times a day to keep us upbeat.

For those who have rough times dealing with a spouse with dementia, I don't want it to seem like we never have hard times. We are just very fortunate that it doesn't make George irritable or angry.

I think impatience and sorrow hit most when I don't get enough sleep. I know that sleepless nights are going to be more frequent as the disease progresses.

I wrote the following after a sleepless night.

Today I am tired and angry.

So angry.

I talk to myself, but logic and reality have no place with this feeling today.

I have seen this in other caregivers. A rage that is under the surface, held in check, and then something happens.

I have listened to some who tell stories of losing it. Ranting and raving and yelling and swearing as they search for the - fill in the blank, keys, wallet, purse, jacket, important document - one more time. Their loved one has misplaced it or hidden it... again. Or they lose it when they have to clean another mess their loved one has created. Maybe it is when they answer the same question for the 20th time.

I have not done that yet. I have not exploded into a ranting rage, at least not at George. But today, today I can feel it coming.

I have observed myself trying to teach him still. "This is the clean dish towel. We only use it to dry the dishes. We do not use it to wipe up the spots in the sink or on the counter or on the floor and you definitely don't use it to wipe your nose." As I talk the logic is like a little person on my shoulder telling me, "Sue, you know this is futile. This is the great un-learning. He is not 4 growing up, he is 69 and his brain is shrinking."

But today I have had *enough*. I hate the smell of shit today.

In the morning he gets me up at 5 a.m. After breakfast I prepare to take him for a walk and I know he usually has a bowel movement in the morning during or after breakfast. So I take him into the bathroom and I ask him to try to go pooh. I set him on the toilet, I hand him a book, and I give him privacy. It doesn't work. He is anxious to go do something. So we go for our walk and when we get back I smell it and I have shit to deal with, and I am tired.

I don't yell, but I do mumble, "This is why I wanted you to go *before* our walk."

A fellow caregiver has a husband that just sits for hours and does nothing. This drives her nuts. I long for times like that.

Today George watches video after video. This week he is no longer interested in coloring or doing puzzles.

George watches movies and that gives me a break to write, cook meals, check email, clean - without him following me into each room. I am so glad to have Netflix and Amazon Prime movies for him to watch.

Another caregiver I know can still leave her husband with dementia for short periods and get out and walk by herself at her own speed.

I shouldn't complain. Ahh no, I have so much to be grateful for. But today, just for today, I am tired, and on the edge of tears, and angry.

So angry.

That day and mood passed. I am feeling blessed again.

Life isn't made of straight lines... but waves. George and I are riding the waves.

My friend Debra has a back injury so I help when I can and visit when I can.

As I write this, George is coloring....

Dementia Care Training and Still Saying Goodbye

August 30, 2017

I should have known.
I kind of knew.
Sometimes I place on the bed the clothes that I want George to put on after his shower. I stay in the shower after I wash and rinse him. He goes out, dries himself and gets dressed.
So when I laid my pants on the end of the bed, I kind of had a nudge in my brain that it wasn't a good idea to leave them there.

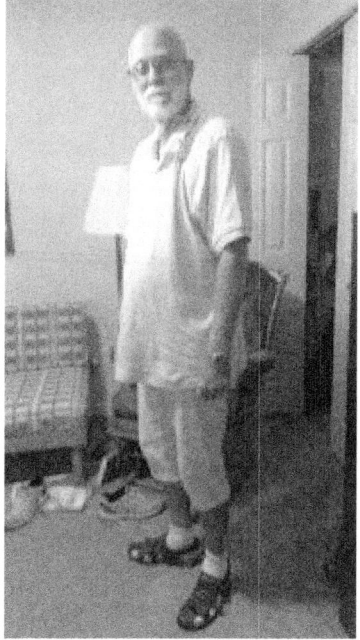

After his shower he put on his bike shoes instead of his tennis shoes. No big deal. When I tell him he has my pants on, the words do not register with him. He just smiles and does his nervous, teary laugh. He wore my pants for the rest of the day.

On Saturday after our bike ride I got him undressed, glasses and watch off, and into the shower. Then, like I have done in the past, I rush to get things ready for when he gets out. I might set his clothes out; I get a fresh towel out and place the old one on the floor. I get myself undressed to get in the shower with him to wash all the places he forgets to wash.

I have to make sure the dirty clothes we take off get in the hamper or he might try putting them back on.

I placed the items in the hamper and turned around and there is George out of the shower already and trying to put his Depends on while dripping wet.

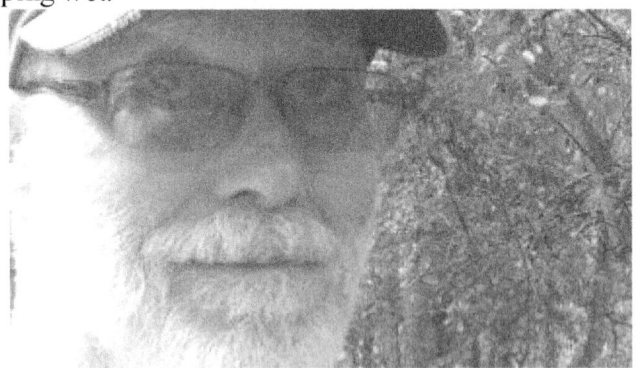

He is agreeable, though he looks at me like I am crazy, when I take him back into the shower to wash his head and face, armpits, butt and back of his legs.

Then a new routine starts: instead of me staying in the shower to wash myself, I follow him out. We are both dripping wet. I dry him off and coach him through getting dressed. I grab a robe and put it over my wet body and take him to the living room. I set him up with a movie to watch. Once he starts watching I keep my fingers crossed that the movie plays through smoothly.

Now I can go take my shower. *Whoo-hoo*!

Caregiver Training

Each time I go to training I come home with more knowledge and a pile of STUFF!!

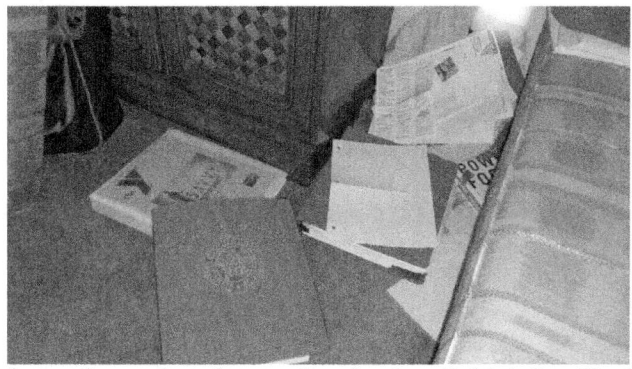

My den is getting quite cluttered and when I think I will clean it, I get distracted with email or phone calls or George saying, "Wanna go do something?"

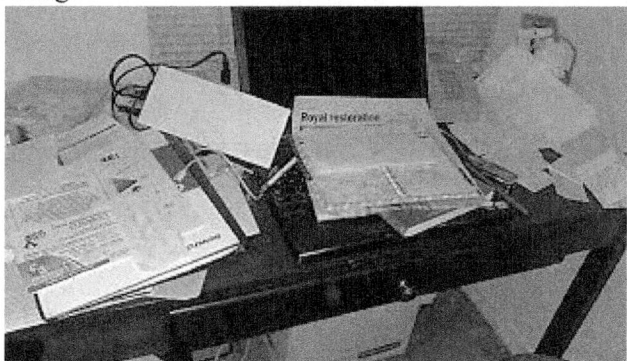

On Friday last week I paid for a day at the Key Training Center so that I could attend a Caregiver Training.

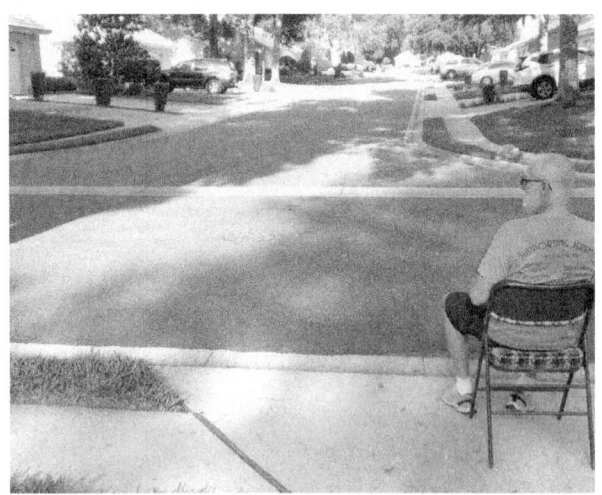

Debbie Selsavage, from Coping with Dementia, spoke in the afternoon and I gained a few tips on dealing with someone with the anxiety or anger that sometimes presents in people with dementia.

A reminder: Dementia is the name for the symptoms and is like an umbrella. Alzheimer's disease is just one file folder under that umbrella. There are about 110 folders under that umbrella. Alzheimer's disease is the one that holds the most papers (patients).

Caregiving Pointers

1) Never touch the person from behind. They are easily spooked and can lash out when surprised. It is better to get in their line of vision (which is narrow). Get your eyes at their eye level and smile. Approach them in a friendly manner. Reach out to shake their hand, but instead of taking their hand, take their thumb pad so you are holding each other at the base of your thumbs.

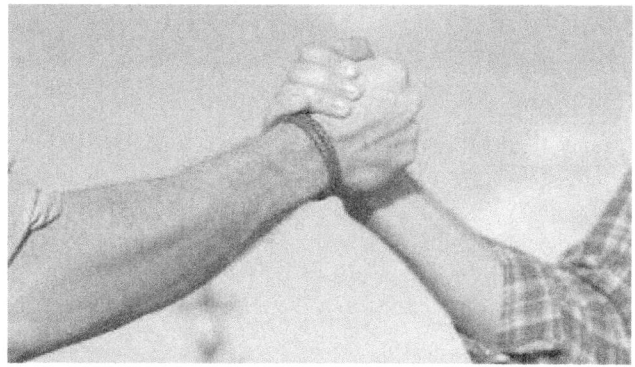

Once they know you and accept your touch, you can keep your hands on them.

Sometimes they can grip but don't get the signal to let go. I have seen George do this when shaking hands with folks. He grips hard and doesn't let go.

2) Enter their fantasy. If they are afraid of what they see, chase that imaginary thing away for them. Empathize with them. If they think someone hasn't come to visit them, and they did visit, just agree, don't argue. Empathize with the feeling.

She said that language is on the left and that the left side of the brain shrinks the most. She said that swear words and music are stored on the right. George doesn't swear... yet. He does like music.

George has lost a lot of his language skills. I usually give him two choices. Sometimes I can tell he isn't choosing, he is "parroting" the words he heard. In that case I choose for him.

I try to keep my requests to one or two words. "Pants, Down... Sit Please. "

A technique I have been using to get him out of the trike is to say "Forward, Forward, Forward" and I place my hand on the back of his shoulder and nudge him forward. So he bends forward from the hips. This takes the weight of his upper torso off his hips so he can lift his hips. Once his legs are almost straight, he can lift the upper torso. Debbie demonstrated this technique at the workshop. Hmmm.

He is still telling people he has dementia. I was on the phone with our friend Jane, and George walked in the room. I handed George the phone and he said, "Hi," and then, "I have dementia," and he started to cry. So he knows, he knows. My poor friend didn't know what to say.

The tears and the thought didn't last long. After the call he was ready to "go do something."

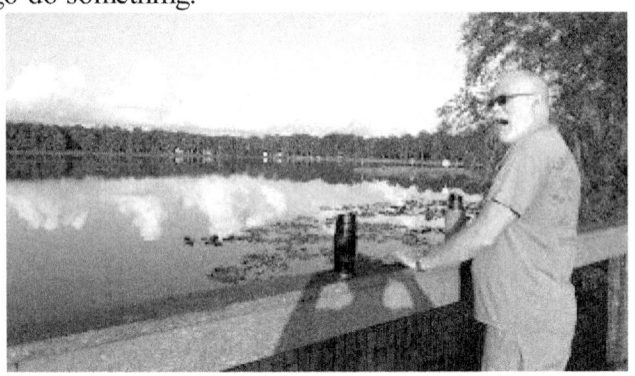

Debbie Selsavage gave out a sheet with "Ten Essentials":

- Never Argue; instead AGREE
- Never Reason; instead DIVERT
- Never Shame; instead DISTRACT
- Never say "You Can't"; instead DO WHAT YOU CAN
- Never Demand; instead ASK
- Never Condescend; instead ENCOURAGE and PRAISE
- Never say "remember"; instead REMINISCE
- Never say "I told you"; instead REPEAT
- Never Lecture; instead REASSURE
- Never Force; instead REINFORCE.

I will add here, Never expect yourself to be perfect; do what you can and take care of yourself.

We all got "fidget mats" at Memory Lane a few weeks ago. A fidget mat is a lap blanket with pockets and zippers and strings, and stuff to fidget with. Even little stuffed toys are attached with a string and stuffed in the pocket. In the late middle stages fidgeting is common and this keeps their hands busy and calms them.

In fact, now I have come to the conclusion that I need something interesting to put in George's hands when I am cleaning him up after a messy bowel movement. It might keep his fingers from spreading the mess. I will look for something plastic and easy to clean.

Work

George stopped doing puzzles recently. Even the 24 piece puzzle seemed too hard for him at times.

Other than TV and coloring, walking and biking, what can I have him do that doesn't require I sit there with him? I started asking around and got some ideas.

Jodie (George's daughter) called and suggested a job for George. There is a video online about a man with Alzheimer's who was worried. He had to get a job. He had to get to work!

So his daughter told him she found a job for him and he would get paid $5 a sheet. She then placed a sheet of bubble wrap in front of him and told him he was to pop each bubble. He was thrilled with his job and spent several hours a day popping bubbles.

I have a case with four rows of different colored poker chips. Occasionally I dump them in a bag and mix them all up and then I ask him to sort them out and put them back in the neat rows in the case for me.

A friend at Memory Lane suggested I take five to seven decks of cards. Mark each deck with a number. Mix the cards up and have George sort them. Doesn't matter if he gets it right, it is something to do. So I am trying that; he has a harder time with that than with the chips. He keeps turning the cards over to look at the face and then getting mixed up. Maybe next time I will have him put all the aces in a pile, all the kings in a pile, and see how he does.

It's All About ME!

Not! However, I have been constantly reminded in caregiver training and in conversations with those who have taken this journey before me to take care of myself. I need to do things that will keep me healthy and will help me find who I will become without George filling my days.

I am trying to do things to take care of me:
- I have started getting a massage every month;
- At least once a week I go to the gym when George has home care or is at Day Care;
- I keep reaching out to friends;
- I study Spanish online most days;
- I do this blog which is not only therapy to see our journey from outside, but it is also something I can look back at and prove to myself that we did the best we could;
- I attend support groups; and
- We do yoga.

Speaking of reaching out to friends, Sunday we stopped in at a friend's and we managed to get George in a kayak that I tied to mine and we went kayaking. I made sure he had a life jacket on. Who knows if he still knows how to swim? We saw three otter, fish, turtles, and birds.

No wonder I have a messy den. Time to get off this blog and start to find places for all the stuff I've got laying around!

Alzheimer's Care Sparks Escape From Hurricane

September 6, 2017

Hurricane Irma is down by Puerto Rico. We have not been through a full-fledged hurricane before. I don't know how it goes, but the truth of the matter is, even the best of the meteorologists doesn't know which way the storm will go and where it will land at this point.

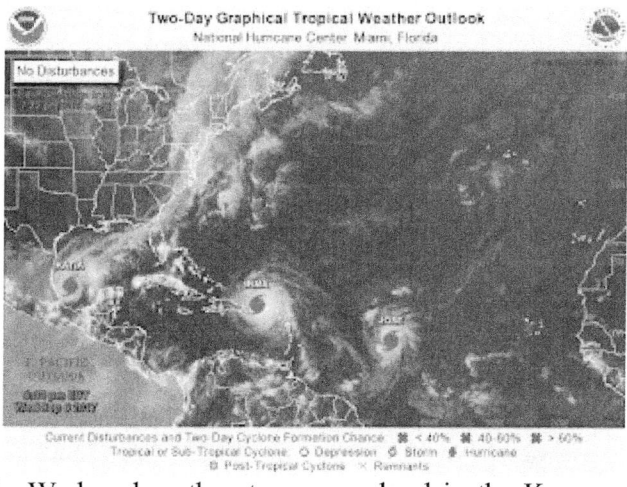

Today is Wednesday; the storm may land in the Keys on Friday, and it may go right up the state. Usually hurricanes get weaker when they hit land. No one knows.

I piled up fresh water just in case and got to thinking about how much water we will need. For a hurricane you are supposed to store four to ten gallons per person per day. Store enough for five days. I use ten gallons or more each time I wash George down after a pooh.

I decided to leave a little water for the roommates and pack up and head north before the roads are bumper-to-bumper (I hear Interstate 75 is already packed and slow).

Yesterday I spent a frustrating hour trying to book a motel in Georgia. Today, while George was at Key Adult Day Care I spent another hour looking for motels in Georgia and calling. Many of them were already booked. I found one half-way, and then one in Rome, Georgia. Rome isn't far from the Silver Comet Bike Trail.

Trikes, luggage, important documents, money, Depends and wet wipes, rags, clothes, extra shoes, umbrellas, snacks....

Oh dang, I just remembered I was going to videotape going through the house and opening drawers so I have documentation of the value and amount of stuff in our home in case... just in case. I hear it is a good thing to have for post-disaster insurance claims. But I forgot. Instead I took the leftovers in the fridge and packed them in a cooler. I made extra ice for the roommates and in case the power goes out. I packed a portable DVD player, George's iPad and mine, but no videos or pictures of our possessions.

As I left town to go pick up George from day care and head out, I saw lines at all the gas stations. George didn't have questions when we started driving up Hwy 19. He seemed relaxed. His hands didn't fidget, he sang along with me and the music I brought along.

I started to think that maybe we should just keep traveling north a bit. Do some trails we haven't done. Maybe even meet up with friends... grand thoughts.

We will see what tomorrow brings.

Anyway, just so "y'all" know. We arrived at our first motel in Thomasville, GA, just fine.

They still don't know where or if the hurricane will land in Florida.

Evacuation Fun

September 7, 2017

We made it all the way to Rome, Georgia. A four-hour drive took us *all* day.

George was a bit fidgety in the passenger seat, but still was good with the travel.

Where we stayed last night, Thomasville, Georgia, has a tree that they claim was an acorn in 1685. We went to see it before we left town.

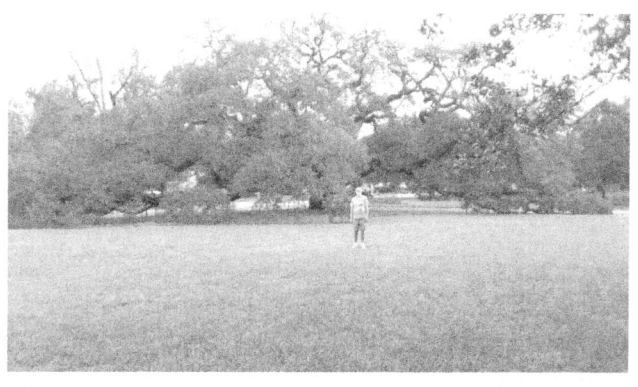

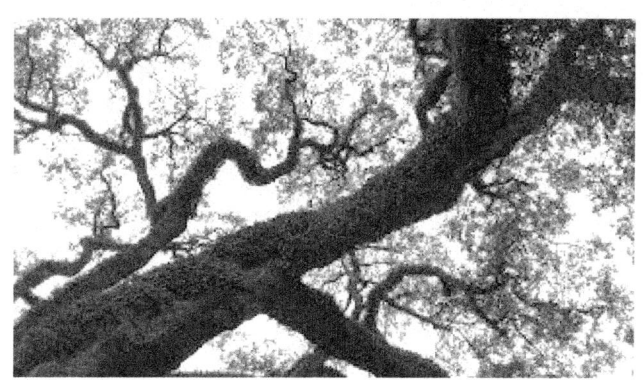

A tree that big and that old doesn't stay intact without some help. Once we walked under its canopy we found cables and structures to keep the limbs and trunk all together.

I stopped for gas. It is 10 cents cheaper and there are no gas lines. George has poopy pants and there is no co-ed toilet. The multi-stall men's is busy. The women's is busy too. I finally go in and ask the women if it is OK to bring my husband into the handicap stall. He needs my help with toileting. They said sure. There was no sink in this handicap stall.

Last week I had got the idea to get false nails put on because my nails were splitting. Now I have strong nails! But, but, "butt" - the new nails hide pooh!

Oh the trouble they can cause! I have to remember to be extra diligent washing; I have even assigned an old toothbrush to the task. These new nails have to go! Rubber glove time!

We found a nice picnic area in Columbus. I was searching for a park when a picnic table sign with an arrow appeared at the side of the highway without warning.

The thing about making a picnic is that I make George's as quickly as possible because he is anxiously awaiting his lunch. Then I make mine. He is done eating before I am and starts eating my sections of oranges and apples. He keeps picking at my lunch!

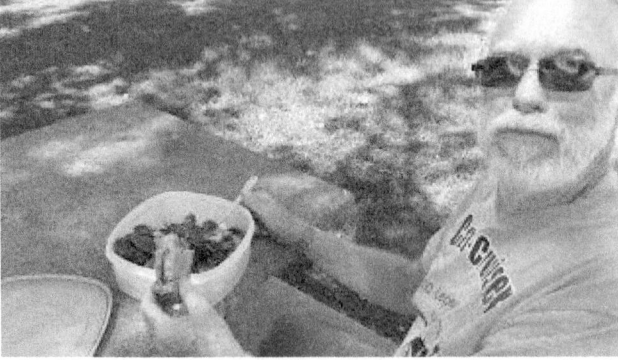

Back on the highway we passed a sign advertising a "wild animal safari." I asked George if he wanted to go see some wild animals. "Ya," he said.

So we went in to buy a ticket and it was $22 per senior! Wow! You drove either a disgusting Jeep or van which you had to rent for another $25 or you drove your own car at your own risk.

We walked away. But first we went to use their restrooms. They looked clean on the surface, actually, but when I dropped my phone and got a glimpse of the side of the toilet, *Holy Crap!*

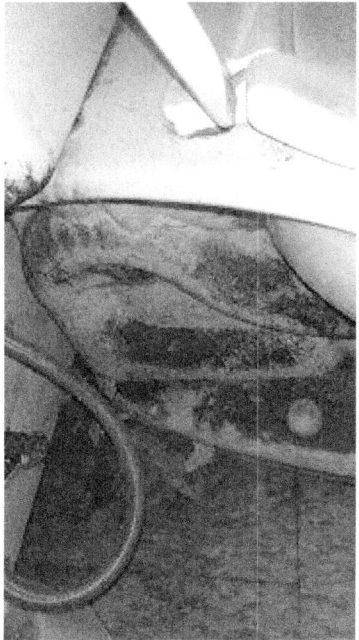

I really wanted to do something different.

I paid the bucks for us to get in and I drove our van into the park.

We did not purchase the cups of food they sell to feed the animals. It is clear that most vehicles do have food. I still have bull snot on my windows.

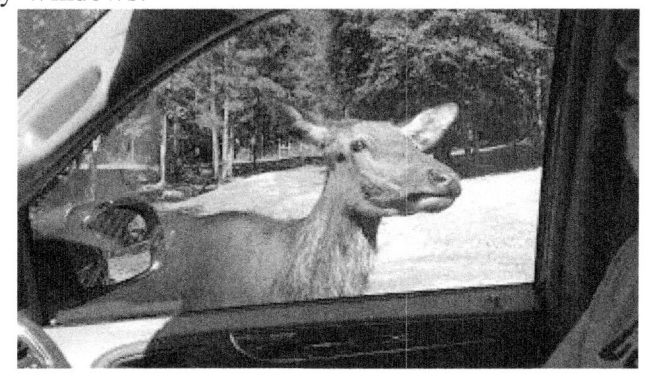

At supper time, we still were not at our destination. George actually spoke and asked if I wanted to stop and get something to eat. We stopped at "Fried Green Tomatoes." It was a buffet with lots of veggies.

Two plates of good stuff and then George had a full plate of dessert. When we got in the car he picked up a bag of chips and started to munch.

I got a text on my phone from the Citrus County Emergency Alert system back home. They have urged voluntary evacuation of all residents of mobile homes and trailers and campers.

It was 7:30 when we finally got to our motel in Rome. I showered George and let him towel off while I showered myself. When I got out he was in his Depends waiting for me. "You can get into bed," I told him. He headed for the door to the motel hallway.

"No, no, no!" I said in a panic. I hear myself say it that way a lot. As if saying "no" one time will not be heard or comprehended? Images of him stepping out into the hall in his underwear were exploding in my head. I guided him into the bed. Then I returned to the bathroom to dry myself off.

I just remembered I forgot to empty the cooler right away when we got to the motel. I did it right now and the ice was all melted. All those wonderful leftovers will have to be tossed. Oh well. As George would have told me, "It is what it is."

Travel Challenges

September 8, 2017

CHALLENGES

We didn't sleep well on our first night in the motel. The plumbing bangs next to our room every time someone turns off their water. Fire doors on rooms and the stairwell were banging all night. Latch click... bang... latch click ....

George and I sat up after trying to sleep and watched late-night TV until after 2:30.

We are at a nice Baymont motel, but the curtain is missing from our room (only the sheer is left to protect glancing eyes from viewing our old, undressed bodies).

The handheld shower squirts out where it is attached to the regular shower head attachment. And when I try to stick the shower head into its holder it doesn't stay, but slides down to the floor of the tub. When I got the repair guy in to fix it, he could not think of a solution other than ordering the parts and waiting for them to arrive. I had him put a screw in at the top so the shower head wouldn't slide down. Then I could take a shower without holding onto the shower head the whole time.

These are small and surmountable problems. They are little challenges that leave this spoiled caregiver muttering expletives under her breath.

After the night of little sleep, I was concerned that George would have a foggy day. He has never been too foggy to bike, but sometimes he bikes a lot slower than others. I had planned on us riding the Silver Comet Trail today. Should we still go?

I know that the storm from the hurricane will send rain and wind this way later this week. We have a window of opportunity to explore this trail.

I drove us from Rome to Rockmart. The car thermometer read 54 degrees! I didn't pack long pants. By the time we got to Rockmart the temp was up in the 60's.

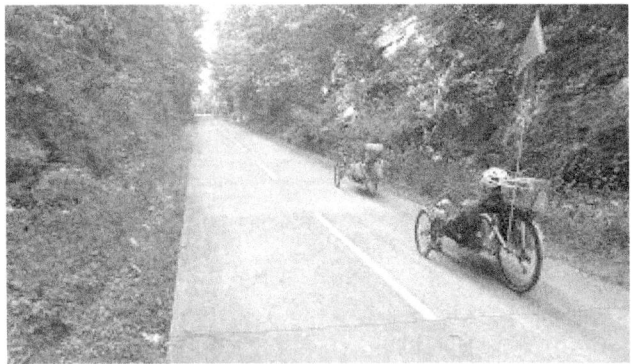

I don't know what the punishment in Florida is for motorized vehicles on the Withlacoochee Trail. I know they have problems with four-wheelers zipping down the trail. In Georgia they don't mess around. You get caught; the fines are big and can include jail time. Florida, take note!

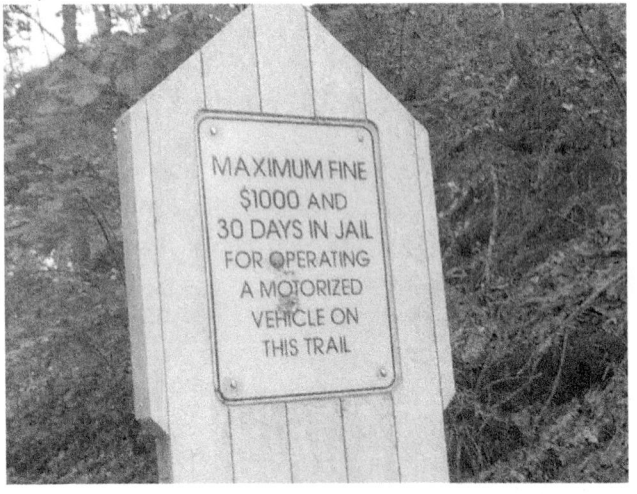

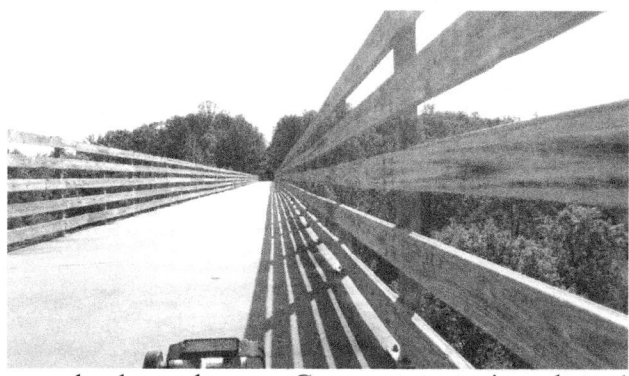

On the way back to the car George was going slow (7 and 8 mph). I kept checking and adjusting his gears. He was not shifting with the hills.

When we arrived at a flush toilet, I went into the men's with him to help him clean up a pooh in his pants.

When we were all done cleaning up I went outside and found several people resting in the area and realized I had forgotten to re-close my trunk and my purse was sitting there for all to see and anyone to grab.

Thank you all good and trustworthy people. My purse was still there intact.

George's speed picked up after he was cleaned off.

In the car traveling back to our motel I took a wrong turn and didn't discover it until many miles down the road.

I punched in the motel address into our car's navigation system.

It kept taking us in the same direction. A long way in the same direction...??? I tried to find a gas station to get a paper map, but (it turns out) they don't sell paper maps anymore.

The GPS was going to take us onto US HWY 41! That highway was bumper to bumper traffic from the people heading north out of Florida!

I made a U-turn and found a Wi-Fi spot outside a Chamber of Commerce. Jodie (our daughter) called just then. I told her I was frustrated and lost. She tried to find a way that didn't put us on 41. But listening to the directions just didn't make sense to me and filled me with dread. It was now after 7 and with no sleep and 36 miles of biking, we were both getting tired.

In frustration I told Jodie we would just head back the way we came. It was a really long way, but I knew the route. And that is what I did.

As we approached Rome, it came to me that George would want supper even with the DQ at 4:30. I had to find a grocery store. A bit nervous about getting lost again, I passed our motel in search of a grocery. I settled for a gas station convenience store where we got ready-to-eat tomato soups and a mac 'n cheese. Now I started to smell pooh again...

We made it to our room!

Only the key didn't work.

There was a line of Floridians at the front desk just arriving after long-long hours in their cars. Thanks to the lady who let me step in and get my key-card re-programmed.

8:30 or 9:00 George is cleaned up again, fed and watching the rest of *Shrek 2*. I texted Jodie to let her know we got back to the motel.

I found a ten-hour sleep sound video on YouTube. It makes the sound of rain on dried leaves. It makes me smile. I will sleep well.

The weather predictions are that even here we will get wind and rain from Irma (2-3" and 30 mph). It is crazy that it would reach this far.

Before climbing in bed, I looked at email and checked the current Irma path predictions. Almost six million people are being evacuated from Southern Florida.

The clerk at Walmart had lived in Florida for 41 years and said it won't hit Florida... she knows, she says, she has watched these predictions all her life.

Debra, my friend in Inverness, stayed. They are ready with a generator, water, grill, food. Still she is nervous and wishing she had left. It is all the media and evacuations that make it scary to stay.

I took the time to look at a map of Rome. There is a bike path down by the river! It looks short, but there are museums and stuff to see.

Roaming Rome

Saturday, September 9, 2017

We had breakfast at the motel and then I worked on the computer a bit and George watched his DVD's. The portable DVD is really saving my sanity this trip.

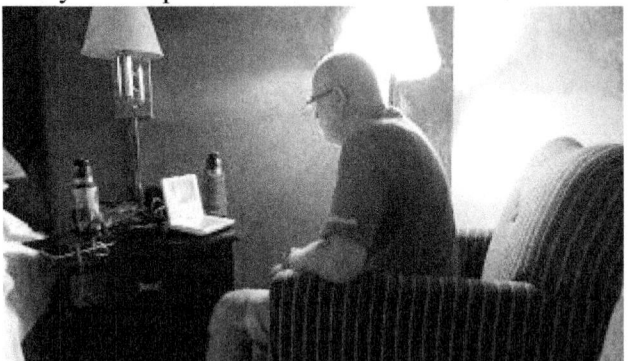

I am checking the weather several times a day to follow the reports and predictions on Hurricane Irma. First, they predicted it was going up the east side of Florida, then a straight hit and going right up the middle, then they predicted it was hitting the west side.

The outer circle of a hurricane has tornadoes that drop down. So even if you are not near the eye of the storm, there can be a lot of damage.

Hurricane Irma is so huge that when it comes by or over the state it will cover the whole state of Florida and parts of adjacent states. It is massive.

In fact, our current location in northwest Georgia may see 50–60 mph winds. I am debating about leaving Rome.

In the morning I took George to downtown Rome to walk around and explore that bike trail I saw on Google maps.

I got George to do a few pushups and dips on the fitness... adult playground.

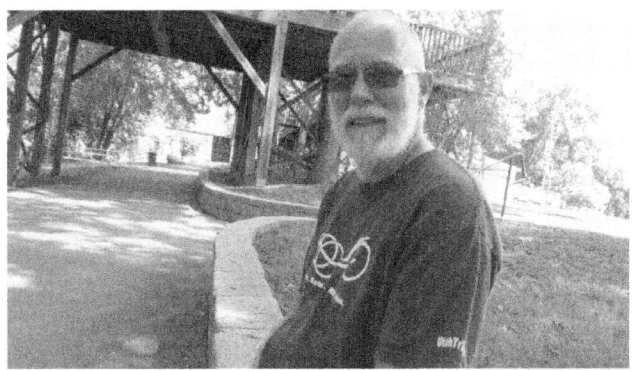

George started to wobble and lean. We sat on a brick wall for a while. As we were sitting a boy (maybe 5 years old) was walking the wall toward us. His younger brother, maybe 4 years old, yelled at him. "Joey, get off the wall! There are humans up there."

Back at the car I pull out the trikes and we ride.

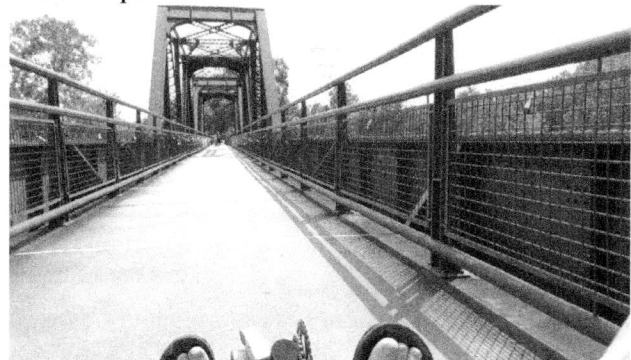

We lost the trail and came to a cemetery on a huge knob hill.... Time to explore.

We climbed some stairs, but then the railing went away. I got us off the stairs and onto a path that spirals around the parameter of the hill getting us closer and closer to the top.

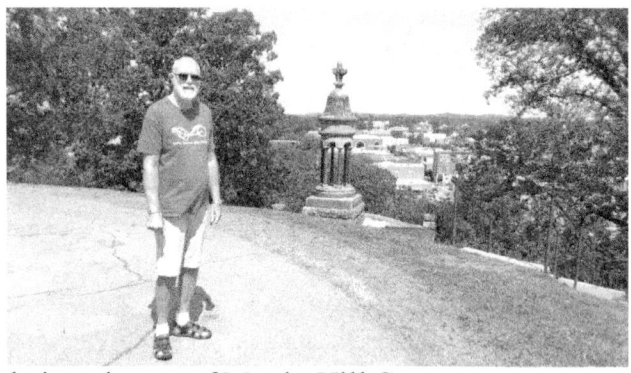

We made it to the top of Myrtle Hill Cemetery.

Civil War soldiers, known and unknown, are buried here.

Back down the hill, we got back on our trikes and went back to the car with only six miles in.

We stopped at a grocery store on our way back to the motel. George watched a movie and I made us dinner. We ate it out in the lobby and met other fleeing Floridians. One guy lives in Naples, and he was in a panic learning that the big storm was headed that way.

After George finished his movie, he wanted to "go do something." I looked online and found Cave Spring.

It is a very small town with a little campground and a big park featuring a spring with potable water.

The storm is to reach our area of Georgia by 8 a.m. on Monday. It is time to decide. Do I stay or do I go in the morning?

Head for the Hills!

Sunday, 09/10/2017

After breakfast we went for a short walk. George is slow and falling behind...

We had a steep hill climb back to the motel and I had to help George get to the grass and stand for a while so he could straighten up and relax a bit. He was losing his balance. He does his nervous, teary laugh.

Back at our room I pulled up a satellite image of Hurricane Irma and decided to head further north. I looked for a place in a forested area in the mountains of North Carolina and the first motel I called had a room for us for three nights for $65/night. I asked about Wi-Fi. No Wi-Fi. I didn't ask about a handicap shower. I figured we would adjust. I just wanted to get further north and east. The storm seems to be heading west once it gets to northern Georgia.

I then looked up thrift shops to find some more DVD's for George. I will need a lot since there is no Wi-Fi where we are going. I also found a laundromat.

George was watching TV and I was able to get us half packed up before he started to want to help. Ha-ha, I spend years training him to stop watching TV and help me do stuff. Now I am telling him, sit down and watch TV please. "The best way you can help me George is to sit and watch TV," I say. A few minutes pass and he picks up two things and stands looking at me.

The motel allowed me to cancel the rest of my days without penalty.

Up in the mountains we stopped at an apple shop. Yes, we bought two apples and two peaches. I then had to use the restroom. George went into one by himself. I went into the other. I always worry when this happens. Is he going to wander away before I get done? Is he going to have a mess?

This time I step out of the bathroom and scan the area for George. He is walking his zombie walk toward the bakery counter. He walks right up to it and of course he can't talk, he has no money. The guy is talking to him by the time I get there. I tell him George has dementia and he is attracted to the sweets. I bought two huge apple fritters. OMG! What am I doing! So much for a healthy diet.

I was delighted when we arrived at our motel and found a fridge and microwave, clean and roomy enough. *And* it has a nice porch and picnic area. As I was checking in I told the owner that George was living with Alzheimer's. He said that he is taking care of his mom (12 years!) and before that he took care of his uncle.

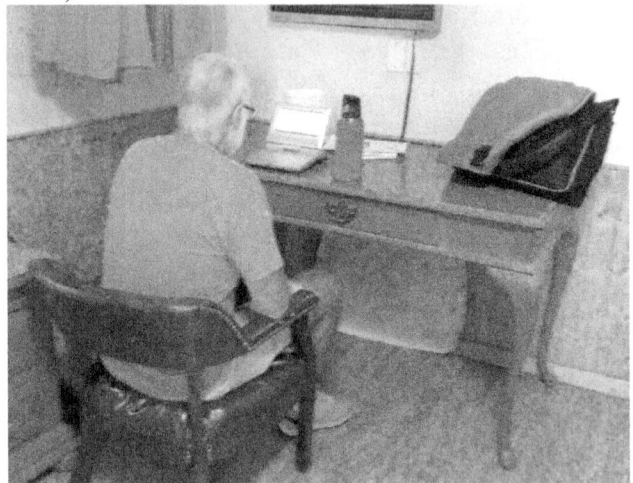

While George watched videos, I made our supper - a huge salad and PB&J. The storm is to hit Inverness now.

Sub-Surface Scream of Frustration

Monday September, 11, 2017

There is no coffee pot in our room; no lobby that offers breakfast. We are in the Smokey Mountains of North Carolina.

I text my friend, Debra, and ask if she is OK and what she sees. We talk on the phone. She slept through it, no damage to her house that she can tell. The power is out.

In Bryson City, NC, the sky is gray and the air is cool. We head to breakfast at the local restaurant and I see a sign for a 9/11 event that reminds me what day this is. Hurricane Irma is still passing through Inverness in the early morning hours; the streets are clogged with debris from trees, and a large area is without power

We walk the streets of Bryson in the early morning chill, and I chide myself for not bringing warmer clothes. I *knew* it would be colder up north in September. The car thermometer says it is 55 degrees. We have only shorts. Fortunately, I did bring our sweatshirts.

I buy a paper to take into the restaurant. But I don't get time to read much of it. George finishes his meal and repeats "Ready to go?" "Are you ready to go?"

I contact a neighbor and ask her to go check on our place and our neighbor's home to see if the neighbor's tree fell on it. She texted back, our home was OK, the tree did fall and damaged our neighbor's home. I was supposed to be watching over their home while they were away. I quickly notified them by phone, text and email. I felt guilty for not being there, though I probably couldn't do much.

Later we stop at the tourist center and get info on thrift shops, the library, and the approach of Irma. Even here places are closing in preparation. Deep Creek National Park has closed to protect visitors from falling trees due to the anticipated winds. Gee whiz! Can't we get away from this thing?

When the library opens I go and set George up with the DVD player and earphones. I was hoping to save our DVD's for later and use the library's DVD's. They wouldn't let us use them without a library card. I gave them a sob story (evacuated Florida, husband with Alzheimer's). Nope. No heart. I blogged as best I could.

We stopped at a grocery store and saw the utility trucks lined up and ready for action in anticipation of the winds expected from Irma. Even here!

I fed us soup in our room. While I was preparing lunch I set George in a chair in front of the TV. He kept standing up. I would ask, "Why did you stand?" He would just laugh his nervous laugh. "Do you need to go to the bathroom?" No. "Do you need to change the channel?" No. I would get him to sit down and then two seconds later he would pop up again. I think he was just hungry. He had a need, but he didn't know what it was.

My neighbor Ken called to let me know about the big tree mess. He seemed frustrated. I tried to tell him it would be a while, since there were a *lot* of trees down and the tree cutters had to prioritize (hospitals, utilities, highways, etc.). While I was talking with him, George picked up the empty suitcase and headed out the door.

I had to call him back three times during my short conversation with our neighbor.

George needed to *go do* something. I decided to drive us to the casino to kill some time. When we got there, I changed my mind and drove 1/2 mile back then I changed my mind again and went back to the casino.

As we were entering we were encouraged to sign up for this card that tracks your gambling and gives you rewards. As a reward for signing up you get $50 worth of gambling credits each.

We had $100 between us to gamble. If that were our money it would be way too much money to gamble. We gamble it and any time we won I cashed out and saved the credits. So we walked out with $30 cash. If that had been our $100 we would have lost $70. But we came out ahead and went out to supper.

I said I wanted pizza. Then I asked George, Mexican or pizza. He said pizza. I take us to an Italian restaurant. On the menu is pizza and also on the menu is lasagna. "Do you want a margarita pizza or the veggie lasagna?" I ask George.

"Veggie lasagna."

We wait. It takes a while. George doesn't speak. I see other couples talking and I wonder what we look like, sitting there, not speaking. We eat bread dipped in vinegar and seasoned oil. We wait. We don't speak. George waits well. I can be grateful he doesn't make insulting comments in a loud voice like some dementia patients. I can be grateful he can sit and wait.

The lasagna comes. He devours his. He looks stuffed. The check comes, I pay, and we get ready to leave.

George says, "We didn't get the pizza yet."

I take him back to our room at the motel. I get him set up with a movie on the DVD player. I text my sister. I am feeling down. No respite care, no way to get away for vigorous exercise which helps my body and mind. I am feeling down because I keep eating the things I know I shouldn't. I am using food as a drug.

I am feeling down as the words of the motel owner sink in. "I have been caring for my mother for *12 years.*"

It is kind of like the coming of this hurricane. It isn't like a tornado; it comes and it is gone. Alzheimer's and many other dementias can last 20 years. The caring gets more difficult. How can I continue to care for him forever? *How can I not?*

Now I am trying to learn to give instructions in one or two words, not long sentences.

For example, when we stopped to do laundry, I told him I was going to put X in the car and I would be right back. He follows me to the car and stands on the passenger side ready to get in.

I repeat, "I am just putting this in the car, George. We aren't going anywhere."

I unlock the car, and he starts to get in. "No, George. No go." I repeat several times.

I put the thing in the car. I close the car and start to walk away. He gets out of the car and follows.

In the bathroom when it is time to change him, I tell him one clothing item at a time.

"We are going to clean you up. Take off your shoes." And if that is too much, I say, "Shoes off... socks off... outer pants off."

Sigh. Sometimes I am energized by what I have learned, the progress. Sometimes I cheer when we get him cleaned up, when we are able to walk a few miles. I have learned to listen to his gait and when he starts to scuff too much I stop him and say, "Look at that straight pole... chest out... heels down on the ground." And we stand a moment and he gets steady. We can walk a while further.

Sometimes I am still shocked and surprised by his disability. I am shocked by his lack of comprehension, his lack of body awareness, the spills on the floor, his shirt and pants.

I am frustrated that I still try to imprint somethings into his memory.

"We are not leaving now. We are here two more nights... George, don't use your butt rag to wipe off the sink... George, don't sit on the bed with your pants off, you may leave a mark.... see???"

Sigh.

I fight tears.

This is just a bump. Tomorrow will be a better day. Our house is still standing; our friends are still alive and unhurt. We are blessed.

A Brighter Day After the Whine

September 12, 2017

I must have slept very well. The motel owner said the wind roared through here. There were several power outages in the area. Irma found us.

We went to a restaurant in downtown Bryson for breakfast and Wi-Fi. I was able to check Facebook pages for Inverness and our home energy company and friends.

We walked in the drizzle after breakfast.

After our walk at George's speed I was looking forward to exercising with a DVD I had found at the discount store. Five miles of walking!

Oh my, what a difference vigorous exercise can do for a person's outlook!

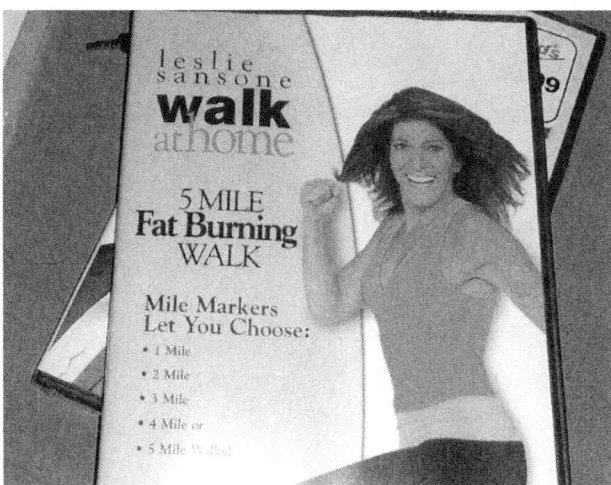

Thanks again to our bike-friend Bill for the wonderful gift of this portable DVD player. What a sanity saver!!

I made lunch in our room and then we went to the library.

George had slobbered toothpaste on his shirt. I didn't care.

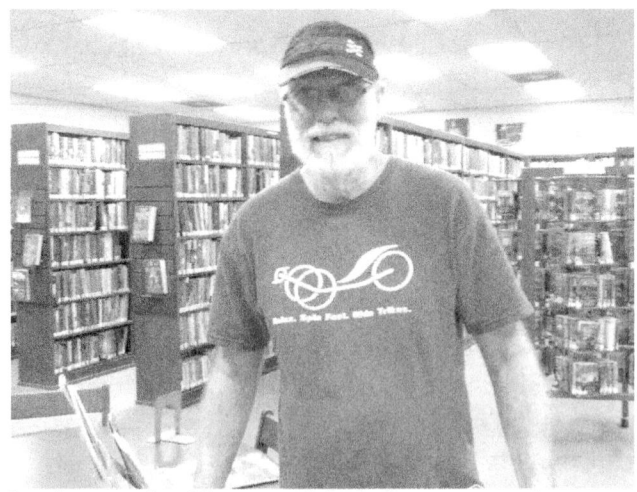

I used the time at the library to blog about yesterday.

Yesterday, the National Park was closed due to Irma's high winds. I decided to drive out there again and see if it was open today. Yes, it was open.

The first short trail was 0.3 of a mile to the first waterfall. It was a steep uphill. I kept an eye on George. I stopped a few times to get him back in balance again.

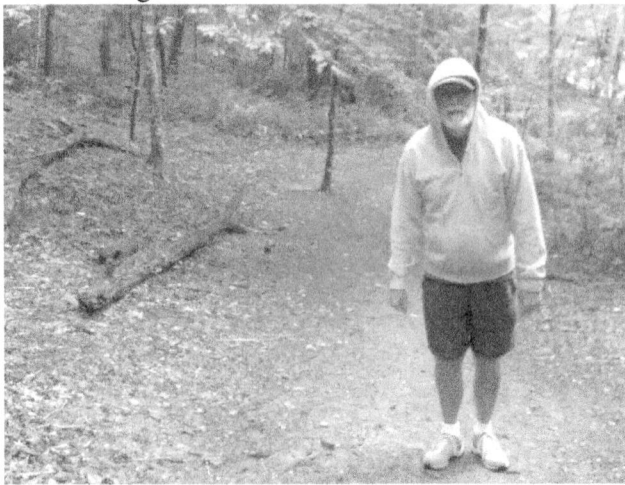

On the way back down the hill, I took his hand and he gripped my hand hard. Once we got back down we took a flat trail to the next falls.

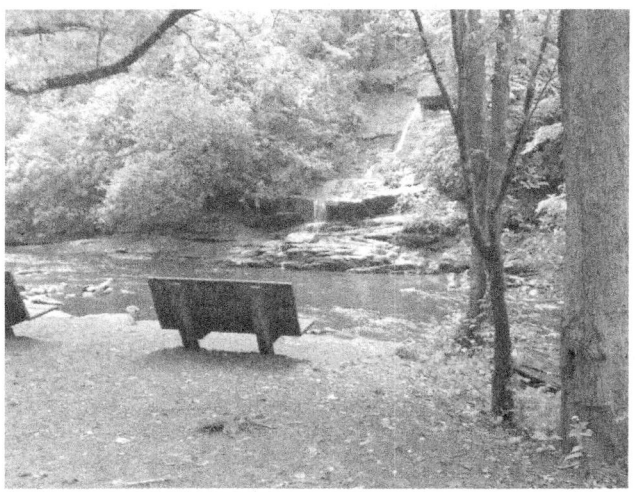

I thought we would sit and enjoy the view for a while. George was only able to sit briefly before he wanted to go do more.

The hand hold is my right hand holding his right thumb. The problem with that is it puts a twist on my spine while I was trying to give him something sturdy to lean on. I tightened my core and hoped I wouldn't feel it tomorrow.

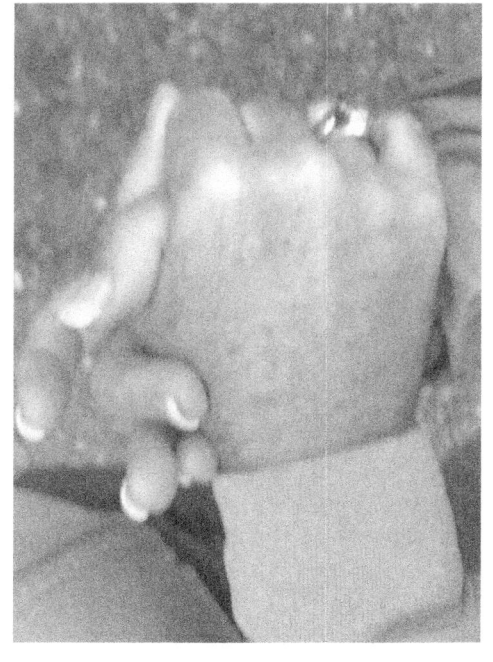

Below is a picture of the downed tree in our front yard. Our neighbor Mari posted it on Facebook. My friend Deb was going to our house today to empty the fridge and freezer for me. She couldn't get in because the tree cutters were there. That is *very* good news. I was thinking it would be many more days before the tree folks arrived to this job.

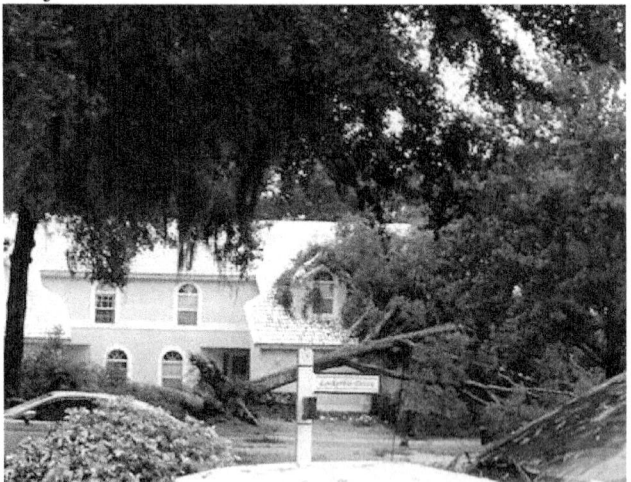

Back in our room I tried to get George to watch TV while I made us some supper. He could not sit for more than a couple minutes. I don't know why... hunger? I would get him to sit down and less than a minute later he was standing up. I fed him and he still was not able to sit. I even put a movie in the DVD player. Instead he was getting up and picking things up like he wanted to pack up.

In the meantime I am trying to decide where we go next or if we reserve another night here. Seeing him anxious to leave I decided to go tomorrow. But where? There is no Wi-Fi in our room, so I go sit down by the office and use their Wi-Fi to look at possible places.... While I am there I see George come out and stand by the car, his hands full of stuff.

The only solution I could think of was to put him to bed at 8:00. He must have been tired. He finally was able to be still. I must have overdone it. We probably "walked" a few miles today.

Surprise! We are Heading Your Way...

The news is that it will take "a long time" to get the power back up in Florida. Is that weeks? Days? I don't know. We might as well take advantage of this travel time and head back to the Midwest to visit family and friends.

Heading out of town we stopped to walk a park and just as we got out of the car we got a call from George's daughter, Jodie! "Hey," I said, "we are coming to visit!" We chatted a while and then she talked with George. He tells her he has dementia. He tells her he misses her and loves her. He asks her what she has been up to. Those are pretty good language skills!

Irma was causing swirly clouds that touched the mountain tops - Smoky Mountains!

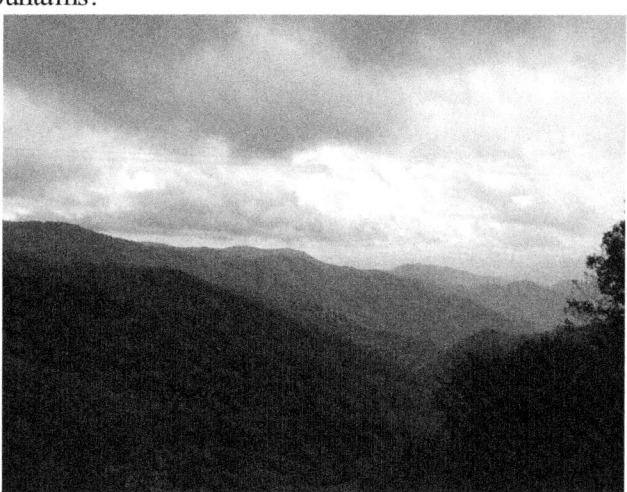

We entered a town with a Dolly Parton waterpark, mini-golf, bumper cars, and a wax museum with King Kong climbing to the top.

I said to George, "This is like Wisconsin Dells on steroids!"
George laughed.

I noticed old cars... on both sides of the highway - for blocks and blocks and blocks.

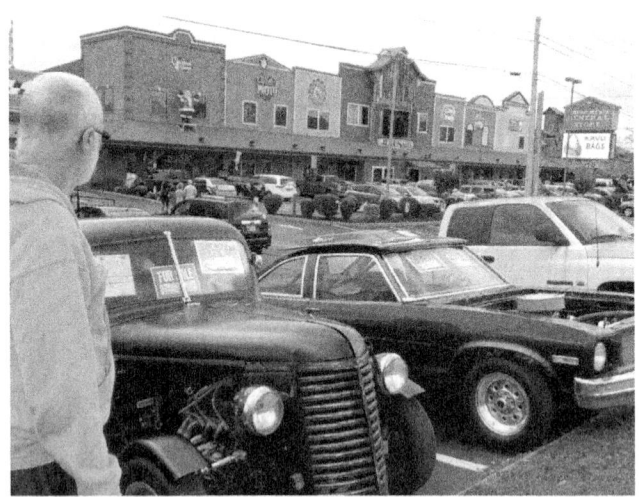

"You want to stop and look?" I asked George.

"Ya," he said fast, without hesitation.

We walked several blocks on both sides of the street. I talked to one of the owners sitting by her car. She said this is a large gathering with old cars the first few days, followed by three or four days of muscle cars. They do this every year.

Further on our long drive we stopped to stretch our legs. It was raining, but we needed a walk.

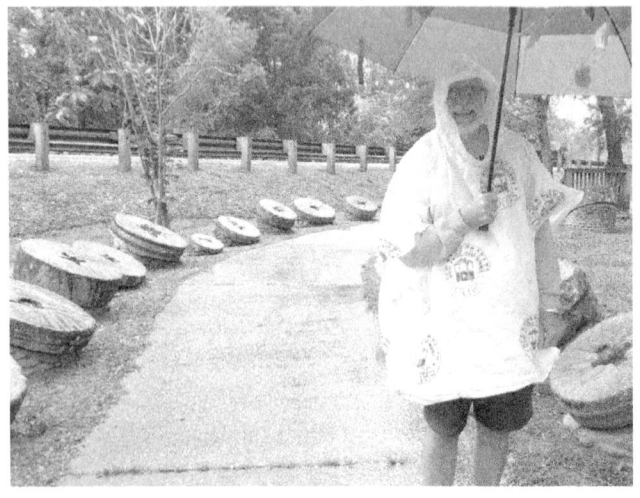

Getting back to the car my sister calls! What are the chances of getting calls on driving days, when I am not driving? It was great to be able to talk and stand watching nature... and begging ducks.

When entering Kentucky we picked up a motel coupon book. We were able to stay at a nice place for $55 for the night. I don't remember where we were.

At home I sleep in another room so I can sleep because sometimes George jerks, and gets up a lot. This room had two beds, which is good. But at 2:30 George got up to use the bathroom. He was changing his pants so I got up with him to make sure he put on fresh pants and didn't fish one out of the trash.

Back in bed, 15 minutes later he was up again to pee. Repeat.

I worry he has an infection, but that doesn't seem to be it. I put sleep music on from YouTube and that helps. He stays in bed until 5:30 a.m. In the morning I smell pee. It is his bed. His diaper must have leaked; that was why he kept getting up. I strip the bed and leave the pile of soiled sheets.

Joy of Traveling With George

September 17, 2017

We had a great visit and stayed with George's daughter, Jodie. Right away on the day we arrived she volunteered to visit with George while I went for a walk and to lunch with my friend from Junior High.

I got in a quick 20-minute walk and then my friend, Bev and I went to lunch. As always, the conversation flowed with Bev. After lunch Bev showed me some of the jewelry she has made.

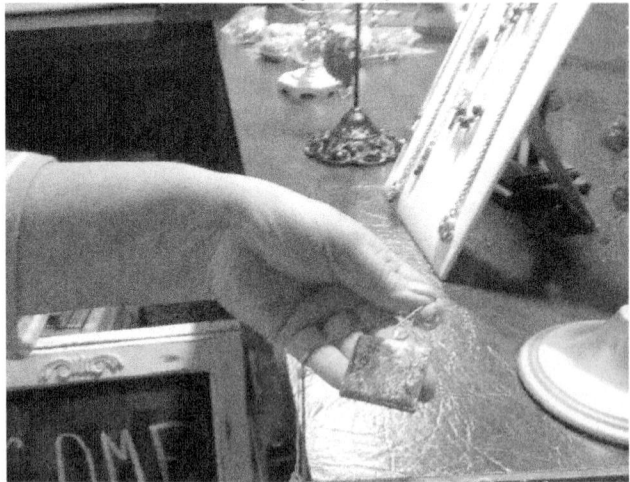

I told her I felt dull now because I had packed just one pair of earrings (the ones I wore) because I was looking for something I could just wear for the five days that I thought I would be out of Florida.

She insisted on making me a set of earrings. I chose feathers to go with a Native-American-made necklace that I own.

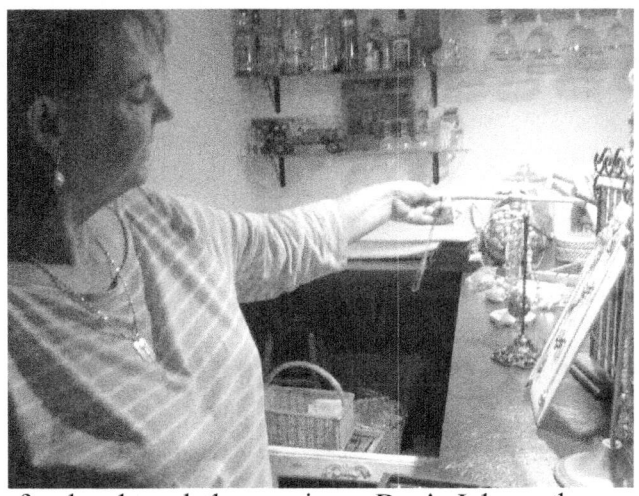

Thanks for lunch and the earrings, Bev! I love them and have been wearing them ever since.

It was amazing how much a little time away from George recharged me.

Jodie had shown George pictures and was happy that George had remembered who she was and the names of her children. She had him help her shuck dried beans. He did well. I said that maybe I could find someone on Craigslist that needs beans removed from their pods. "Free labor available."

I took George with me to get the oil changed in the car.

Then we both got haircuts. $45 with tip.

George got real foggy toward the evening. He did not comprehend simple phrases or words, and he didn't respond when we spoke to him. He had a lot going on interacting with Jodie all day. He'd used up all his brain energy.

At night he was up four times or more to go pee. We were in the basement and I was afraid he'd be too unstable to climb the stairs at night. So we used the laundry tub and I rinsed it down. It worked and was a safe alternative.

One time his bed was wet and I had to change the sheets.

On Saturday, Jodie and Carl took George along with them on some errands and I got to relax and go for a fast walk.

Later in the day they took us to a flea market. Every time Jodie would ask George how he was doing he would tell her, "I got dementia." She would say, "I know and I love you anyway," or "That's OK." Once she said, "How's that going?"

George shook his head with his teary laugh. Awwww.

George kept telling her he loves her and looking at her with adoration. It was sweet to see.

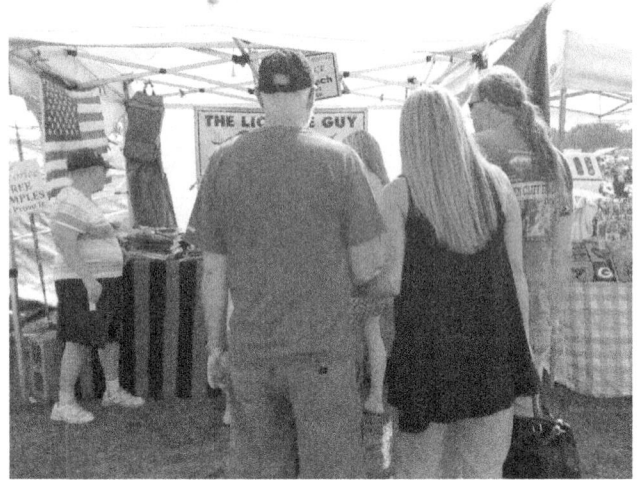

At the market, George was shadowing Jodie.

All the things to look at were kind of overwhelming for me. I remember hearing at a caregiver conference that grocery stores can be very difficult for people with dementia. George didn't show any signs of anxiety.

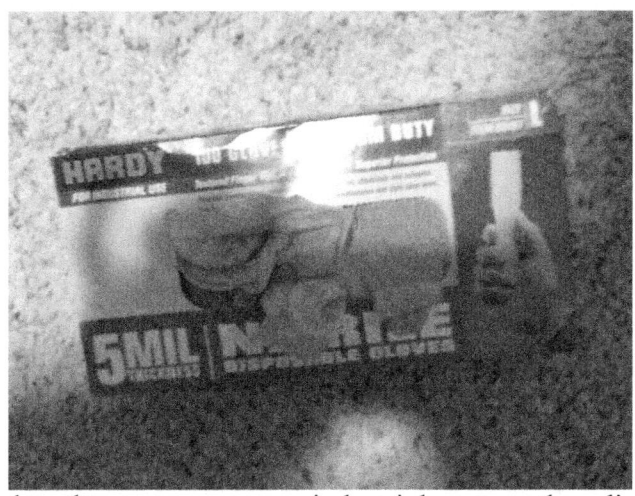

Jodie bought me some industrial strength disposable gloves! They fit well and my fake fingernails don't poke through. They need to make them go up to about the elbow though. Sometimes it's that messy.

While running errands, Jodie got me some disposable mattress pads to use. This will come in handy on our travels.

On Sunday morning George had a particularly messy pooh. It took a while, but I got him all cleaned up and sat him on the couch to watch a video. Later in the morning Jodie pointed out the back of his pants were stained.

I took him back in the bathroom and realized I had forgotten to check to see if his shorts had gotten messed up and had him put the same shorts back on. They were a mess on the inside. Jodie is resourceful. I am sure she will figure out exactly what to do to clean her leather couch where he was sitting.

Now I will use the disposable pads when I am visiting someone.

After a nice morning at Jodie's, we headed for Waukesha which is 90 miles away near Milwaukee, WI.

The drive was very pleasant. The fields have turned golden; a few trees are hinting at reds and yellows against dark greens. Lovely.

We stopped in Delavan and I picked up some buns and cheese and asked the clerks at the grocery store where we might find a park with a picnic table to have our lunch. The cashier didn't know anything about parks, but the bagger named off three parks and gave me directions to Springs Park.

I had some pesto that I spread on the buns with the cheese. The sandwiches were yummy.

George said he pooped again. "No problem," I said. "We will find a bathroom with water and take care of it."

But it turned out to be a false alarm. That is good, too.

We went for a walk, did some pushups and dips and found some slides big enough for us.

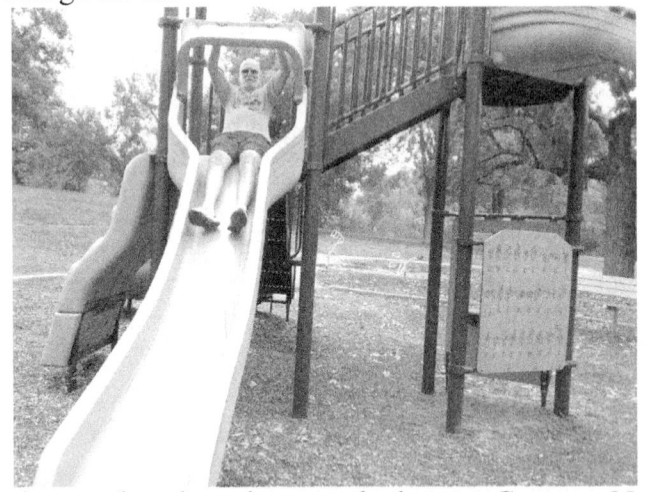

I have always played at playgrounds, but not George. Now with the left side of his brain shrinking, he is able to have fun at the playground too. I took a picture that makes my heart sing; George is just coming off the slide with a big smile on his face.

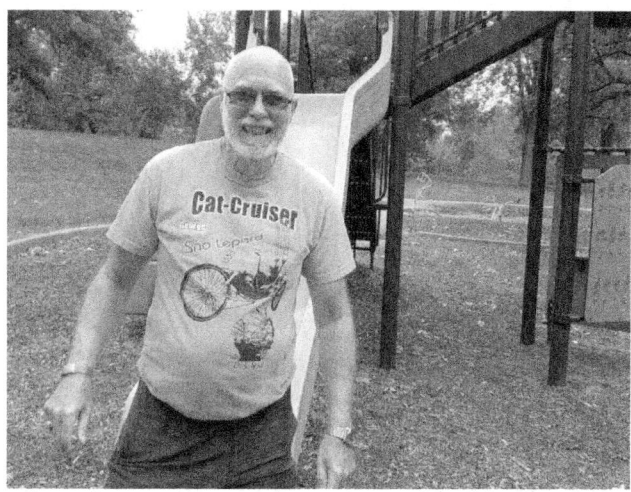

Instead of saving money and staying with friends, I decided to save my nerves instead and stay at a motel. What a relief to pull things out of the suitcase and put them in drawers. To know we are going to be here three nights, and not have to worry about smells, seepage, or over-staying our welcome.

It was time to wash clothes again already. The motel had guest laundry facilities. George watched *Colombo* on TV and I did laundry.

After dinner I drove us to Waukesha's Frame Park and we walked the path around the lake.

Back at our room we showered and I set George in bed with pillows to watch an episode of *Love Boat*.

More work on the computer takes me way too late into the night. Tomorrow we are meeting our friends Mark and Jane and riding on the Glacial Drumlin Trail. Yahoo!! Let's ride!

Beautiful Fall Day

September 18, 2017

What a beautiful, cool, fall day. It was great for biking with friends, Mark and Jane, on the Glacial Drumlin Trail.

We were to meet our friends at the E.B. Shurts Building trailhead at 9 a.m.

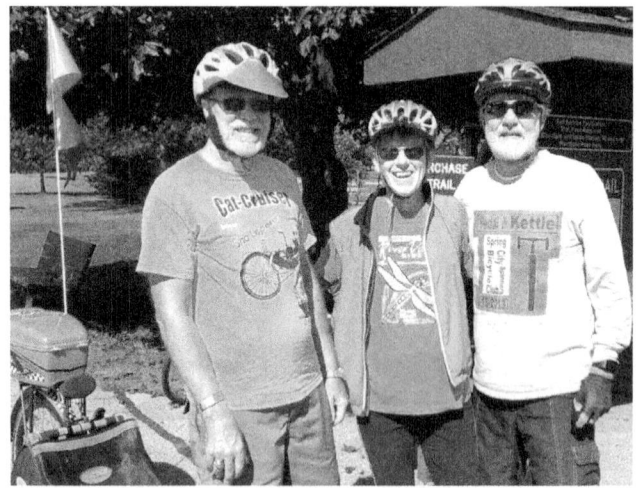

It was lovely seeing our friends again. Jane gave me an awesome hug, and I felt the tension drain from my shoulders. Then we rode up the trail. We pedaled past bunches of bright wild asters, pretty Queen Anne's lace, and cornfields turning golden.

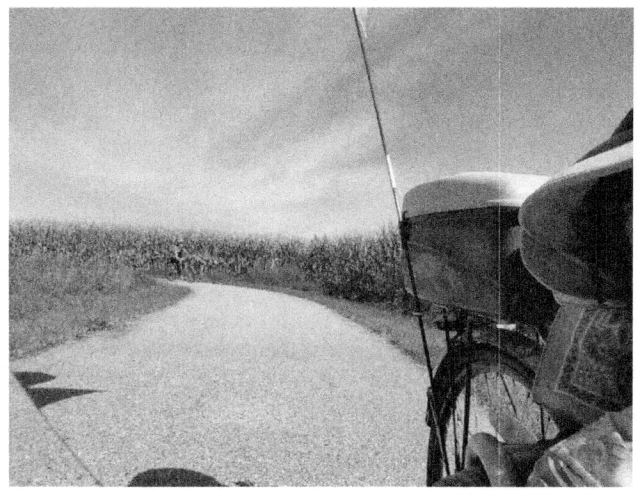

As we were getting ready to load the bikes, George's legs started to shake and I had to direct him into the car to sit. This is a new symptom I haven't seen before. Mark helped me load the bikes in the van.

Back at our room George watched more TV, and I got news that the Withlacoochee State Trail in Inverness had opened up for biking after the storm. Great news! I plotted out the days for the rest of our trip. It was time to think about what needs to be done before we return home.

I sent out an email to our bike group to let them know the trail was open again after Irma.

At 4:30 we went to visit our son Jeremy and his family. Jeremy has chronic illnesses that still have no definitive diagnosis or cure. He was very bloated with water retention. He's been in a lot of pain and discomfort.

Jeremy poked his finger into his shin and showed me how the dent remained.

We left after just a short visit because Jeremy was feeling awful.

Tomorrow I hope to bike a different trail. We have plans to visit our friends Sandy and John.

Great Days Full Of "No!... Don't... Stop!"

I yelled at George in our motel room. I apologized later, but I yelled and I got rough. That happened later in the day. Most of our day was great. Great weather, beautiful rides, fantastic food and friends. It was a wonderful day.

In the morning we biked from Sussex, Wisconsin to Menomonee Falls on the Bugline Trail. It was about 62 degrees and lovely.

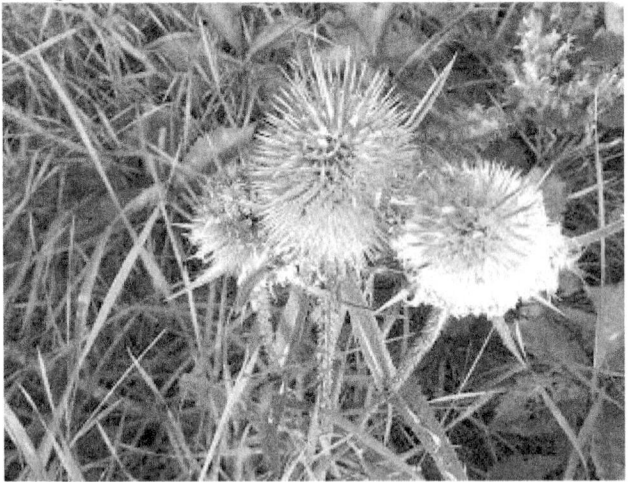

George can no longer get out of his trike on his own. Later in the day he can't get out of chairs by himself. He can no longer scoot his chair up to the table without help.

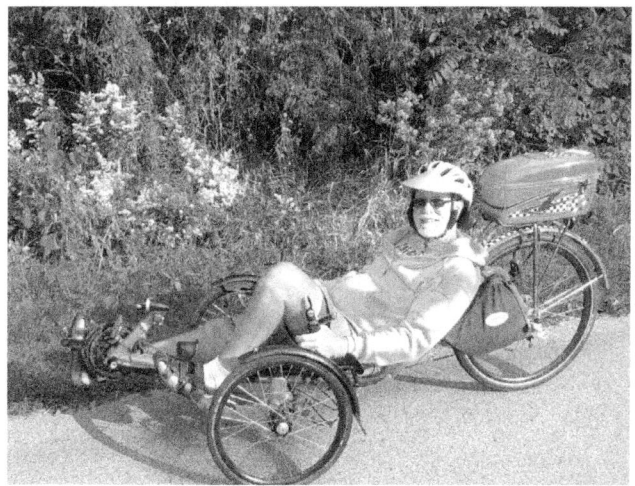

At noon we went to Sandy and John's home in Sussex, Wisconsin. Sandy is a gardener and her garden was happy this year.

She cut a lovely head of red cabbage for me to take.

For lunch she started us out with a kale and banana smoothie followed by lots of veggies from her garden. Yummy! I am sooo grateful for the great friends in our life. Thank you, Sandy and John!

After lunch we pulled the bikes out again to ride more of the Bugline Trail.

I was getting my bike ready to ride when I turned around. George was sinking into his trike with difficulty. We get on the trikes by stepping *in front of* the crossbar. George had, for the first time, stepped *behind* the crossbar. Getting him out of this wasn't going to be easy.

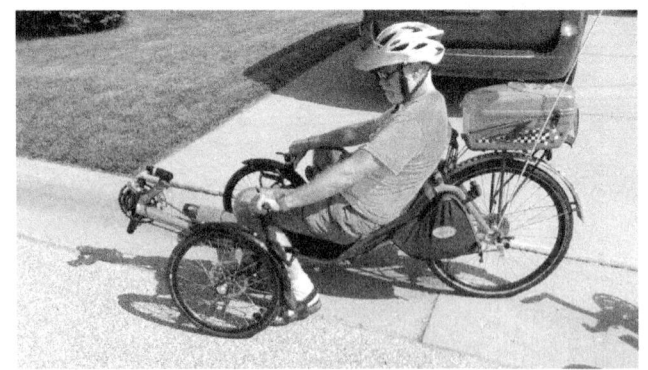

He isn't limber enough to put his knee up toward his chest to move the leg over the crossbar.

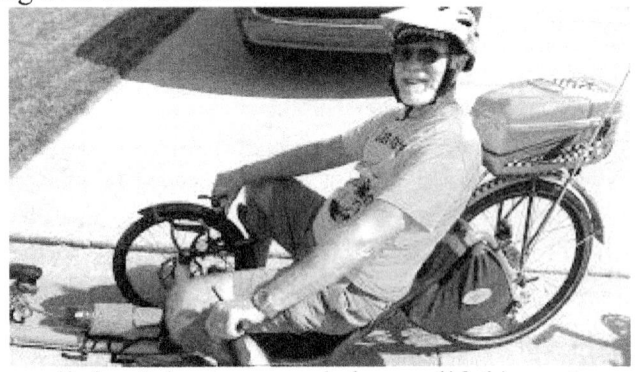

I had to call for John to come help me lift him. As we lifted, George knew enough to pull his leg up and move it over the crossbar. Yeah!

After a lovely ride and more visiting, George and I went back to our motel room so I could clean him up and get ready for dinner over at Mark and Jane's.

We get in the motel room. I go to the bathroom and check messages on my cell. When I come out of the bathroom, George has my computer and all the wires from our electronics sitting on the bed with the computer case.

"What are you doing, George?" I ask.

"G g g getting ready to go," he said with a big smile.

"We aren't leaving," I tell him. "We are here another night."

I guide him into the bathroom to brush his teeth. I get him going with toothbrush and toothpaste and guide him to lean over the sink. But he doesn't lean much and dribbles on the floor and the counter.

As he is going at it I head back to the bed to put the wires back on the electronics, but he follows me brushing and dripping. So back to the sink we go and I stay until he has rinsed and dried.

Then I get a text from my sister to check my email.

I turn on the computer and George goes back in the bathroom and comes out with our cosmetic kit.

"No, we aren't leaving, George. Put that back," I say.

He returns to the bathroom and comes back with his toothbrush and toothpaste in hand.

"No, put that back in the bathroom. We aren't going anywhere," I say.

He goes back in the bathroom and while I am reading and responding to the email George returns twice more with the cosmetic kit. I smell pooh.

I ask him to come into the bathroom. I tell him to take his shorts off. He un-snaps and un-zips and then re-zips and re-snaps. We go through this twice more. We remove his Depends, and as I turn to the waste basket, he leans his butt against the wall so he can reach down and put the new Depends on.

"Hold on," I say. "You have a poopy butt. Let me clean you off."

I step around him to get the wet wipes and I have to remind him to "Hold on, don't move" a few more times. He wants to put on the clean Depends.

I finally grab the clean Depends and throw them on the floor. "NOT YET!" I say. "WAIT A MINUTE!"

I grab a washrag and while I am at the sink, George leans his butt on the door jamb to bend over to pick up the Depends.

"NO!" I yell. I put my foot on the Depends and kick them back out of the room. "NOT YET! Now you have poop on the door jamb! Just be still. We have to finish cleaning you up!"

And then I scrubbed his bottom vigorously. I return to the sink to rinse the rag, and he starts reaching for his shorts. Well, dang!

After he was cleaned up and dressed... I sat him in front of the TV and tried to get myself dressed between putting things back when he picks them up to pack them.

I then hugged him and said, "Sometimes this is challenging. I am sorry for yelling."

No response from George. No kisses to my neck, no I love you. Sigh, I think I upset him. Does he remember I yelled at him? Does he remember or know why? Did my yelling remind him of his decline?

No time to discuss, we leave to go to Mark and Jane's for dinner. She has made a wonderful Ratatouille (thank goodness for spell check on that one!) and a lovely salad. She gave me a light beer and I *really* enjoyed it. Just what I needed; good friends, good food, good conversation!

Mark showed us his baby fish in his fish pond. He showed us some of the great photos he has taken and pictures of their granddaughter. Such a cutie!

At 8:30 I am tired and we head back to our motel.

I sit George in front of the TV with some popcorn. And I check email and start to write this blog. I see him nodding off to sleep so I get him ready for bed, tuck him in. I hug him and he says, "I love you."

A few minutes later he gets up, heads into the bathroom. I follow. He has removed his Depends and dug a soiled one out of the trash to put on.

Then he is peeing on the floor. I clean him and the floor and put him back in bed.

I sure hope he sleeps well tonight.

Fortunate Encounters

September 20, 2017

Travel Day today. I got George to watch a movie, at least for a little while, so I could get packed. When I was about finished, he started moving, so I had him go with me to the lobby to get ice and back to the lobby to get the cart.

The drive today was *lovely*. The early autumn colors were unbelievably beautiful.

Our first stop was in Madison, Wisconsin, to visit our good friends Kathi and Karl. Kathi is also a caregiver - to Karl, who is living (and sleeping a lot) with dementia. When we arrived, Karl was sitting and sleeping, but stirred when we walked in so I went and sat next to him and said, "Hi Karl, it's Sue Straley."

He smiled and said, "George!" as he looked around the room and found George. George came up and they smiled and shook hands.

Karl has always been thin, but now he is like a walking skeleton. He doesn't like to eat much.

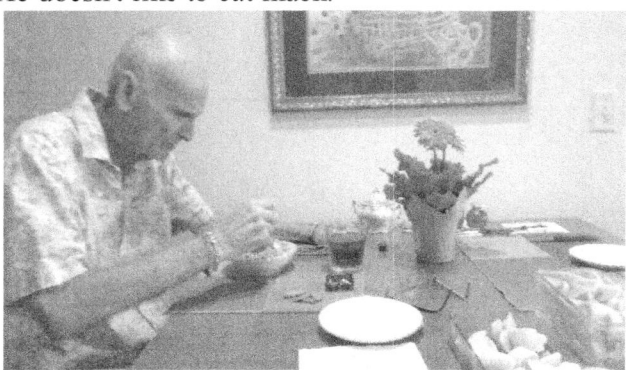

Our mutual friend Kay had sent George a fidget spinner a while back. (It has survived several cycles in the washing machine and is something I can hand to George when he is anxious.) Kay sent Kathi some napkins with three ants printed on them... life size. They look 3D and real. Karl and George were trying several times to kill those ants. Smashing them with fingers and spoons and folding the napkin over and smooshing some more. Karl was even giggling.

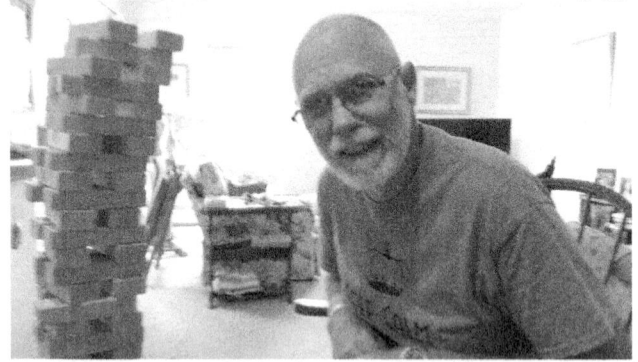

Kathi brought out a wood-block game and George stacked them all.

It was wonderful to visit with Kathi. She is an awesome person and friend who has been through a lot in her life and is still dealing with it with courage and grace.

We leave there and head north toward Rhinelander, WI. We are scheduled to arrive by 6 p.m. My sister Mary has a pot of chili waiting for us.

We needed a break so we stopped in Stevens Point at a shopping area and walked around. We came upon a nail place and I had my fake nails removed. I had them give George a pedicure; $66 with tip.

We are now here at Mary and Dave's home on the river.

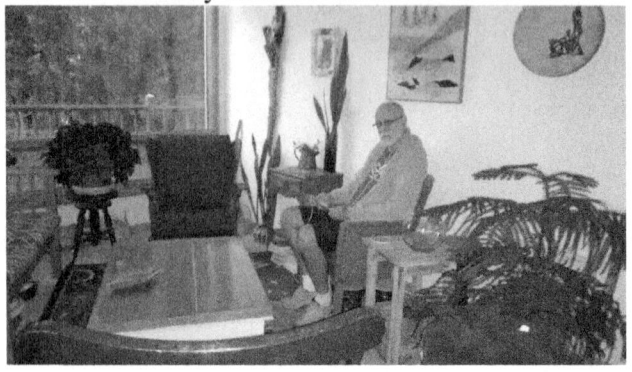

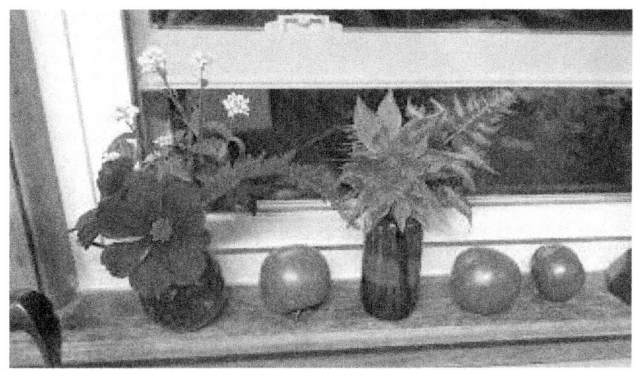

Mary had graciously emptied drawers in the bedroom and provided space in the bathroom for our stuff so we could settle in and not live out of our suitcase. Our toilet supplies are like a fungus spreading over the surfaces of their bathroom.

We dine over chili and then George and I are both yawning.

I check email and several friends are suggesting we return home. They say that routine is good for Alzheimer's disease. Other patients, and maybe George, will do better there. I know that George is doing the same on the road as he does at home. His dementia has been progressing all year and the new behaviors or loss of ability I have seen on this trip is really in line with what I have witnessed at home.

Some have suggested it is time to put George in a home. And though I would love to have a full overnight break or several days' break, there are some factors that keep me from doing that.

1) I can't afford it. Memory care costs $3,000 to $4,000 a month.

2) As long as I can get some respite care and sleep at night I can keep doing this.

3) George is still a travel companion, a presence in my life. As long as he is here, I am still part of a couple. I still love him... most of the time.

4) I don't want to give up control of his care - such as when he gets his soiled pants checked and changed, how much exercise he gets, etc. I guess I still care very much about him.

But yes, we will be heading home... after visiting my sister and checking out a few more trails.

Sleep-Deprived Caregiver Grumbles

September 22, 2017

When I don't get enough sleep, my attitude as a caregiver stumbles and rumbles and grumbles.

George and I exercised to videos in Mary's back yard. First we did squats, lunges, and pushups with Chris Powell and then yoga with Rachel Scott.

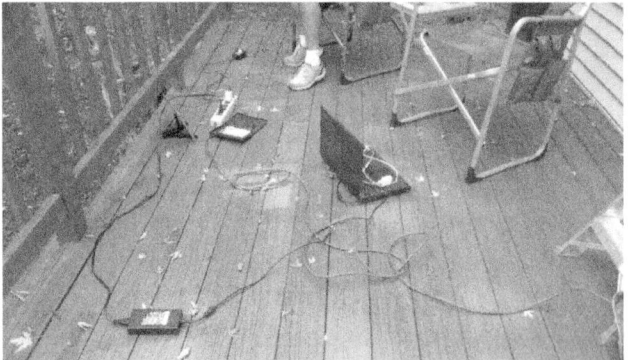

I made us lunch and did laundry (George's Depends leaked again last night).

When Mary returned from work, we all sat on the back deck. I set George up with his DVD. The first one he didn't seem to want to watch, so I put a different one in.

I was tired and aching. *Had I worked out too hard?* I wondered.

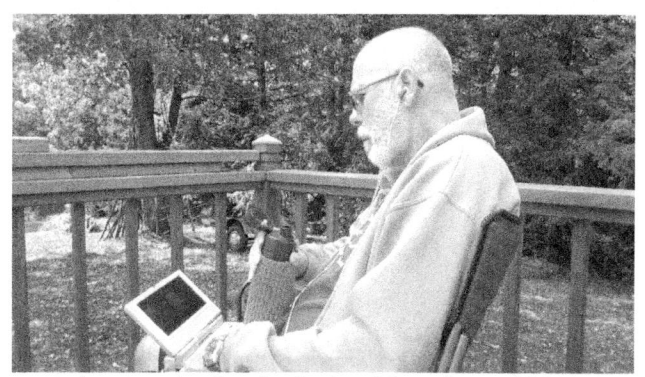

We were sitting on the back deck. It's a beautiful spot. Autumn colors touching the leaves, the breeze flapping through the sheets on the line. I decided to lie on the deck and nap.

I was there two minutes at most when CRASH! I jumped. George had stood up and dropped the DVD player and it fell into two pieces.

I grabbed the pieces from him. "Why can't you just settle down and give me some time to rest!??" I growled. At the same time I was saying it, I was silently scolding myself for acting like a spoiled child. Of course, he isn't being bothersome on purpose. He is doing the best he can with what he has. And, of course, life is good, and I am being a bit too grumpy for the situation.

Mary jumped into action and convinced George to follow her to walk Spirit, their dog. Thank you, Mary! She is always thinking of ways to make it easier for others.

Fortunately, the DVD got put back together and still worked. While they walked, I felt in a rush to get my "chill" on... to relax my tense body and mind before they returned.

After wandering around a bit wondering what I should do with this precious time, I went and sat on a rock by some lavender and garlic in the back yard and just watched the insects working and the leaves floating on the breeze.

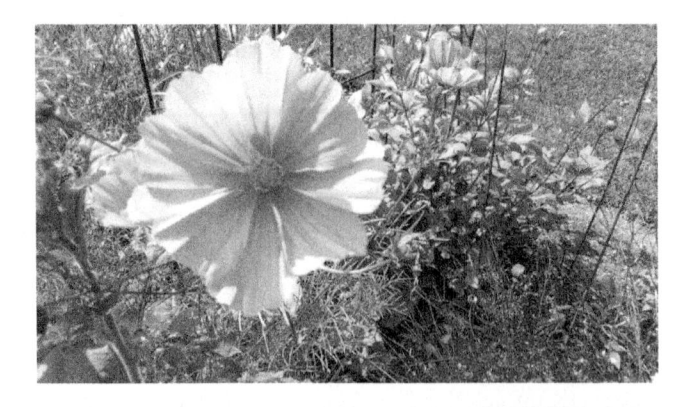

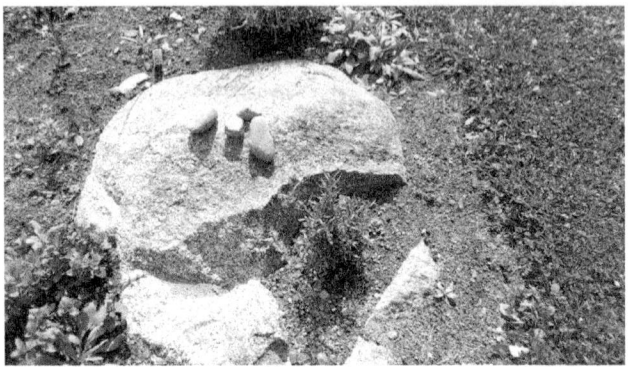

When Mary returned, we talked about getting respite care here, but the day care places would require doctor's notes, and that may take days to process my application. Mary called around and found a woman who does companion services. She arranged to stop over on Friday at 4:30 to meet us and arrange for some respite time on Saturday.

Mary had made wonderful veggie lasagna that she put in the oven for dinner.

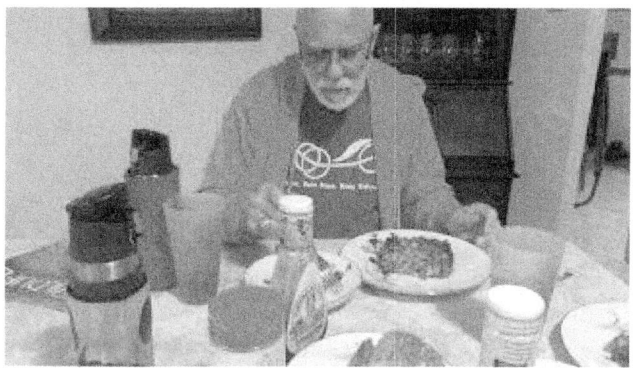

After dinner George started packing stuff whenever I got busy with not watching him (like going to the restroom myself).

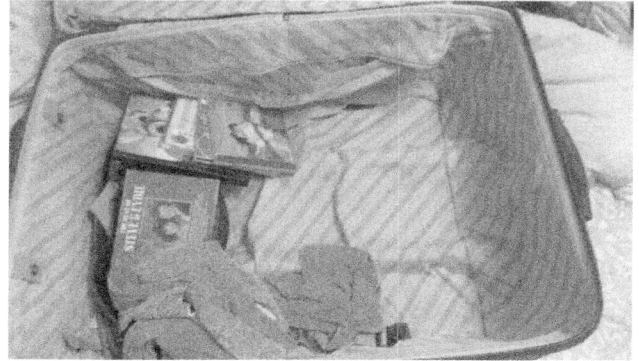

Thursday night, George only got up once to use the bathroom and I slept well. Hurray!

A Peek into George's Sorrow

Saturday, September 23, 2017

    The caregiver who was going to provide respite for me canceled and it was just as well. We had decided to go over to Boulder Junction, WI, to ride the trail. Riding and caring for George after sleeping well is no problem.
    After breakfast, George and I took a short walk. George hovers too close.

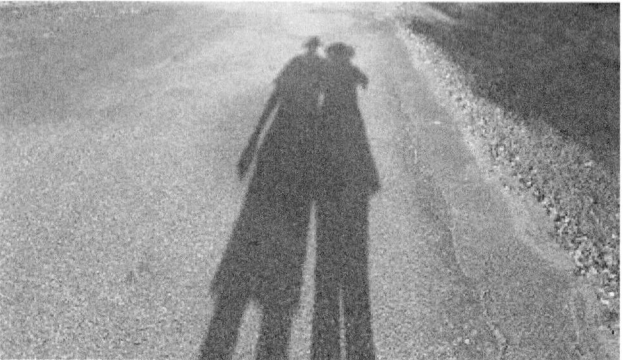

I create some space for myself. Like my new hat?

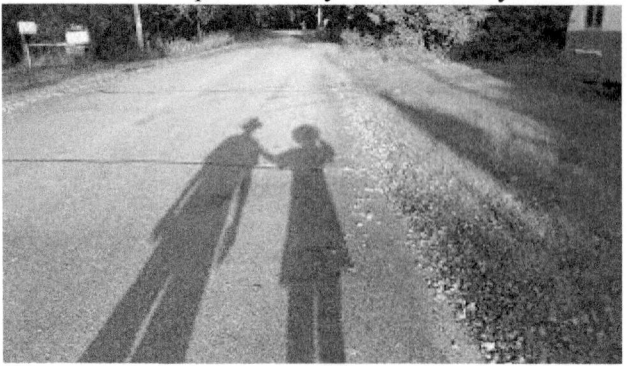

    We passed these plants. Mary calls them Cup Plants. The plants cup water at the base of their leaves.

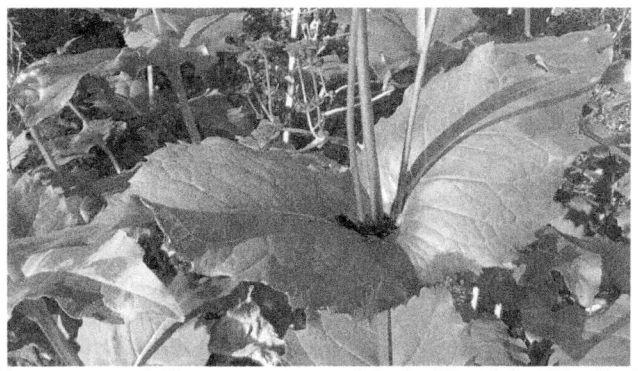

The trail we were riding connects with the Boulder Trail. It is called the Manitowish Waters Trail. It is paved and curvy with hills. We rode 11 or 12 miles to a park in Manitowish.

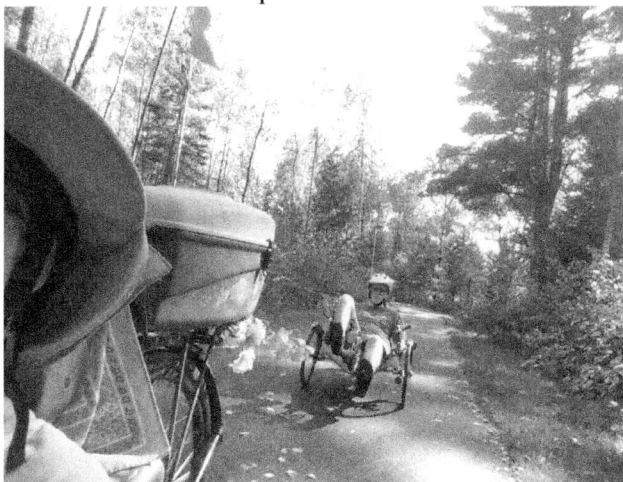

It is unreal to have an 86 degree afternoon again and again this late in September in northern Wisconsin.

We had a picnic lunch at the park in Manitowish.

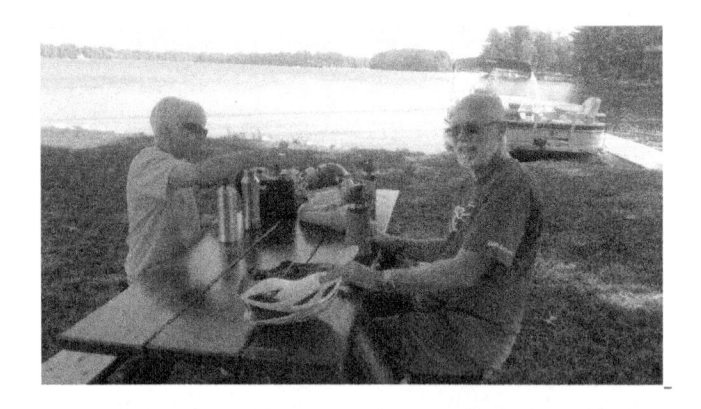

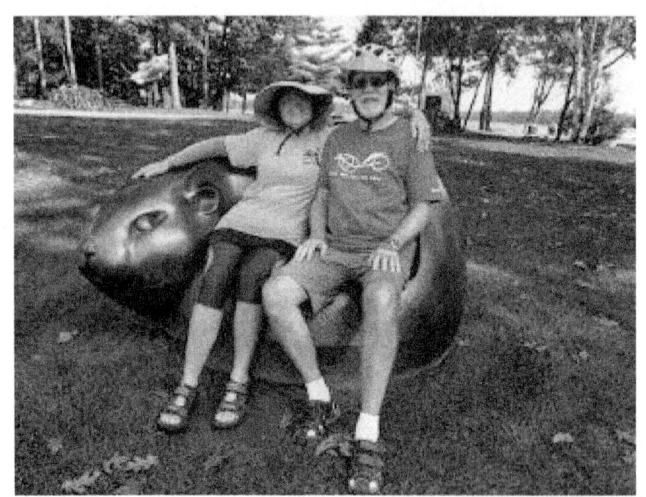

I only had to stop and push George up the steep hills twice. He did pretty well.

When we pulled back into the parking lot this is what I saw...

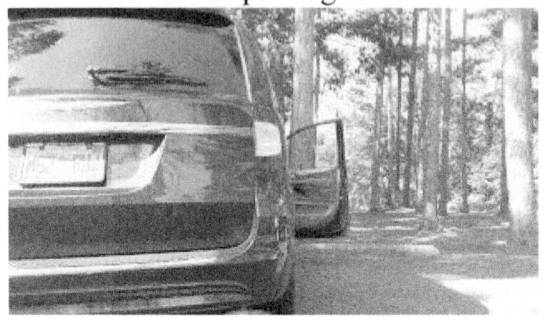

I had left the door open on our van! Nothing was missing. Wow!

I told George to sit in his trike and relax while I unpacked my trike and put my shoes on. He didn't say anything to that, but his face said he wasn't happy about it. He can't get out of the trike without my help. He scooted his trike up so I couldn't get my trike in the van. I asked him to scoot back, and he either ignored me or didn't want to comply.

Mary intervened and told him she was moving his trike back and would help him put on his shoes, which she did while I loaded up my trike.

I helped George get up, and he went and sat in the front seat without trying to help me put his trike into the car.

When I got in, I saw that he wasn't smiling at me, and he had looked less happy today. So I asked how he was doing. He looked sad and teary and shook his head.

I kissed his shoulder and told him I loved him. I told him he is doing well for what he is working with. I told him he rode well today.

I have heard that a caregiver's go-to solution to behavior and mood problems in those with dementia is… ice cream. We stopped in Boulder and got ice cream.

On the way back to Mary's, I searched for a park with flush toilets to clean George, but didn't find any. When we arrived back at Mary's, she greeted us with a cheery greeting. I directed George right into the bathroom without stopping to chat.

Then we all sat out on the deck for a while before dinner. The deck looks out over the yard and the river. On this lovely fall day it was a beautiful and relaxing view.

After dinner Mary had the fire pit all set up with citronella candles, chairs and the fire already started. I couldn't imagine a better sister. Thank you!

Up Over the Lake - Mackinaw City

September 24, 2017

    I got myself and George dressed. We were on the road again.
    We turned north on Hwy 41. It hit me that this was the same US Hwy 41 that goes right through our town of Inverness, Florida.
    But instead of turning south toward home, I turn north.

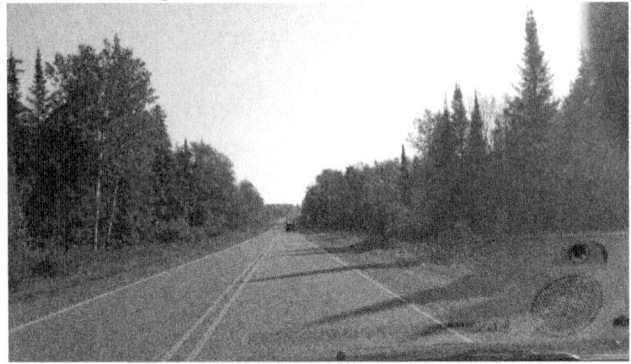

    Most of the waysides along Hwy 8 in Wisconsin were closed... budget cuts. I stopped at a wayside in Michigan.
    I tried to stop every hour or so after lunch to stretch our legs.

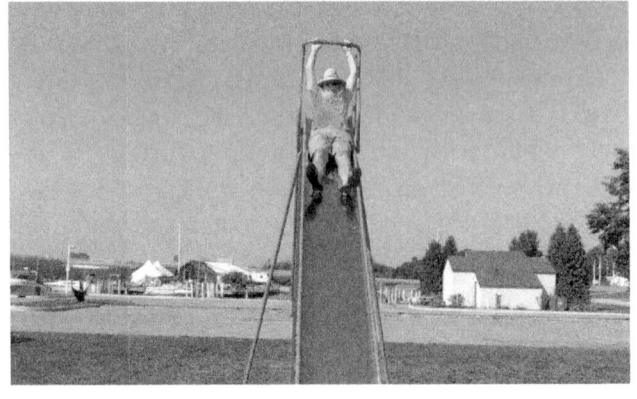

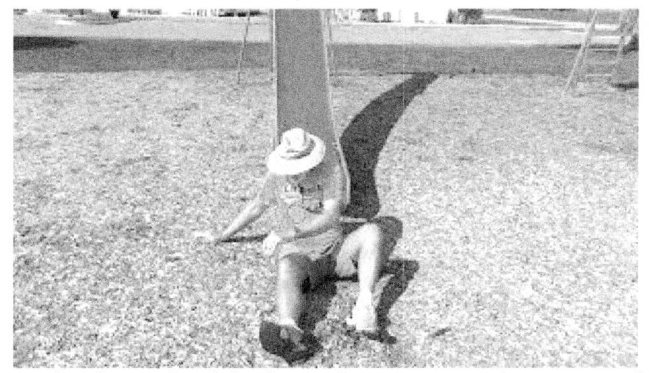

On this path along the lakefront there was a sign post with signs giving the distance to cities.

It turned out we were about halfway between Seattle, WA, and Pensacola, FL! I thought about it for just a quick moment. *Nahhh*, I said; we are heading home.

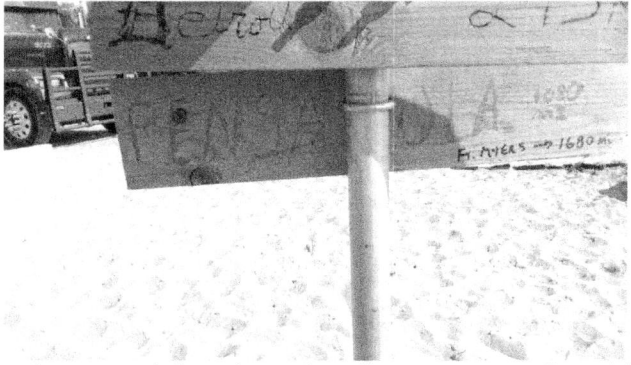

We paused on a park bench to give George a rest. I could tell the walking was getting more difficult for him.

On the walk back to the car he tripped on a bump in the sidewalk and ran forward. I was ahead of him and grabbed his hands as he went by, and that helped him catch himself before he fell.

I then gave him my hand to hold, but instead of doing right hand to right hand which stresses my back, I had him hold my left hand. He held it very tight the whole way back to the car.

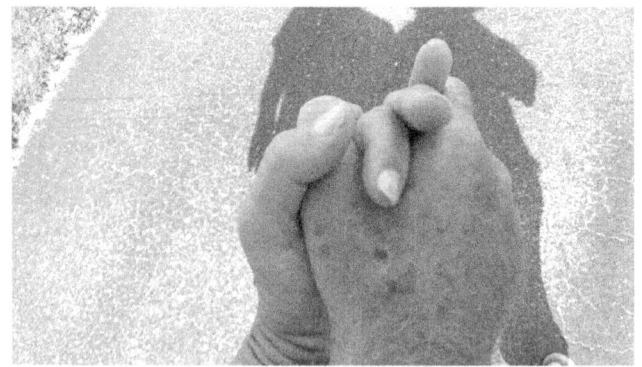

After crossing the Mackinaw Bridge into Mackinaw City, I parked in the touristy downtown area by the ferry. We walked down to the ticket office and bought the ferry tickets we will use tomorrow to go to the island. We have never been to Mackinac Island.

Then we made our way back to Dairy Queen, passing up several fudge, taffy and popcorn places on the way. While ordering the blizzards, I got a whiff of pooh.

While we ate our ice cream, I called the Rainbow Motel I had found on Google Maps. Price was $53 the first night and $50 the second night. Nice!

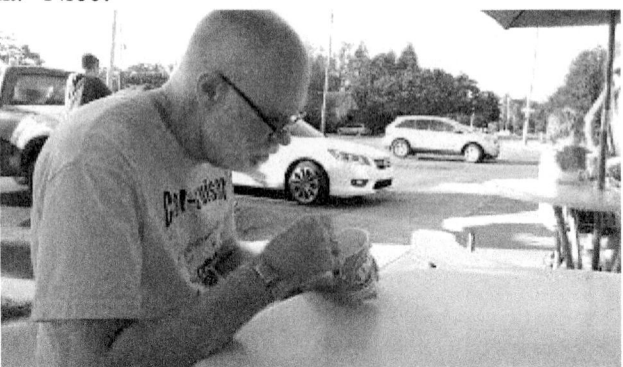

Mary packed leftover lasagna for us! So we had a delicious supper in our room.

A caregiver needs to read labels carefully. I discovered the last batch of Depends that I bought were not "Maximum Absorbency." The Max provides fewer leaks at night. My sister also said that some Certified Nursing Assistants will add two women's Maxi pads to the inside of the pants at night time to avoid spillage.

I also learned I bought the wrong kind of wipes. These are nice, but they are not flushable. Not a problem as long as I am aware and can plan for it.

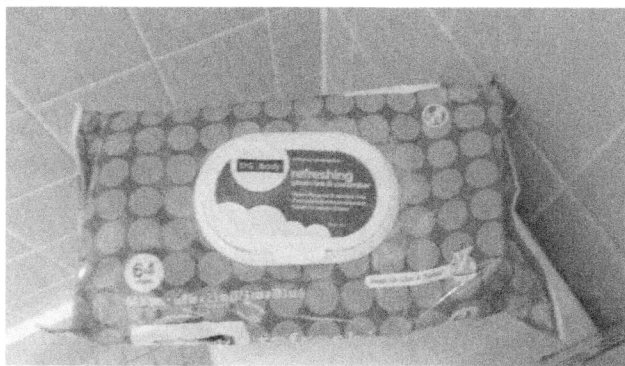

Mackinac Island

September 25, 2017

Today we took the ferry to Mackinac Island.

At breakfast, George was sad. I made an extra effort to be cheerful and helpful today.

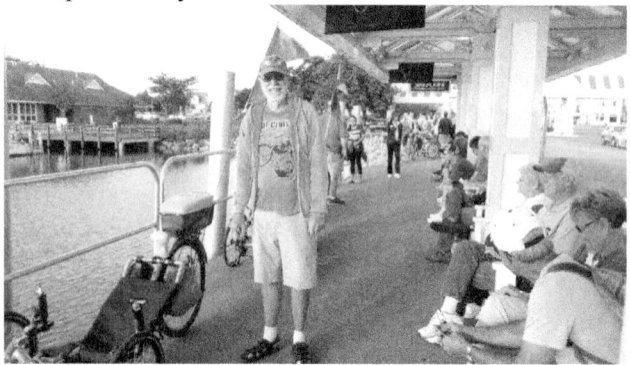

Lake Huron here is crystal clear. We can see the bottom... but no fish, no turtles, and certainly no gators.

We waited in line for the ferry, watching people and a cute little dog wearing his PJ's.

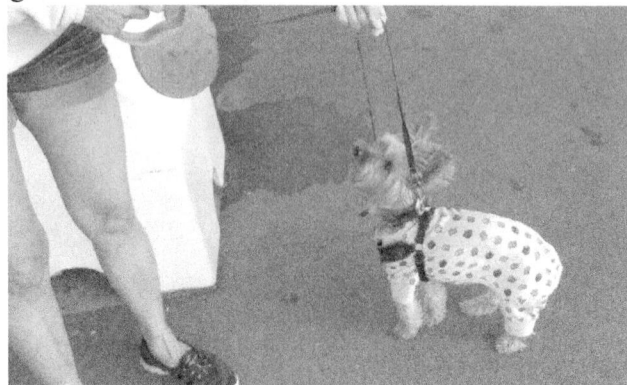

It turns out the 9 a.m. ferry takes a little detour under the Mackinac Bridge.

They are painting the bridge constantly. By the time they get all the way across, they have to start over. Five miles is a *lot* to paint!

Mackinac Island has no autos, just very *big* horses and lots of bicycles.

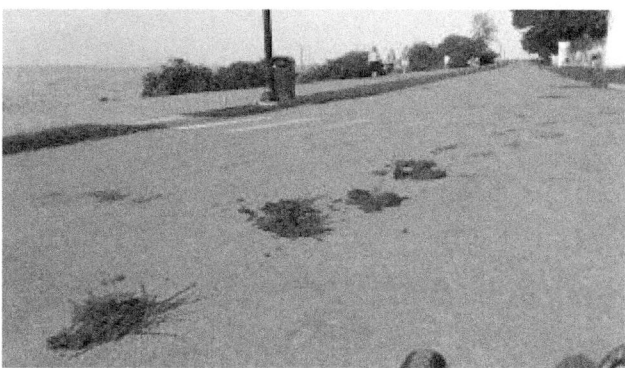

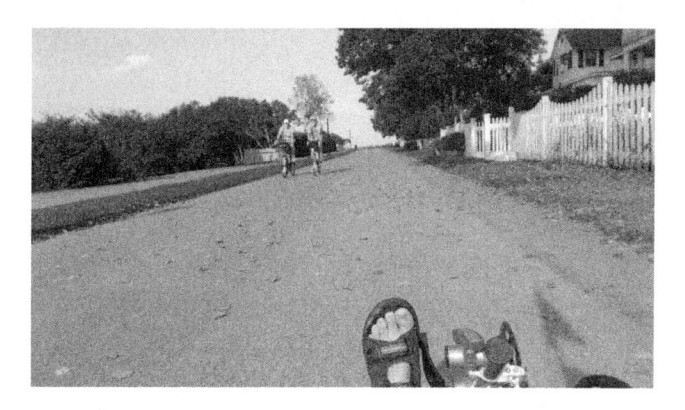

We rode the perimeter trail three times. I stopped in town and tried to see some things but the hills were hard for George to walk. A friend urged us to take the carriage ride; $29 per person. I didn't want it that bad.

Back on the mainland we stopped at the shop by our motel that sold pasties. A pasty is a folded pie crust with meat and vegetables inside (or, as in our case, just vegetables like potatoes and turnips).

We sat at a table to eat our pasties. I ran out to the trike to get my phone. When I returned to our table, I noticed that George was still wearing his bike helmet.

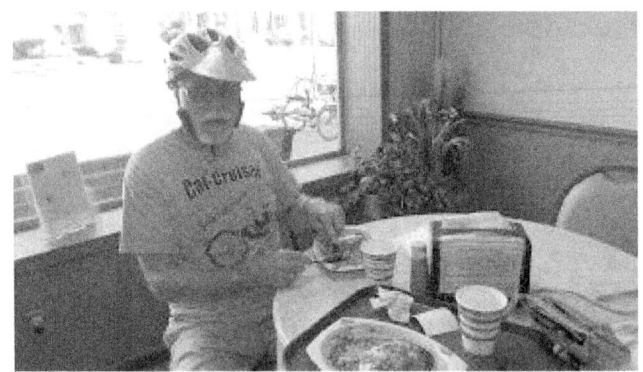

This evening I am careful not to start cleaning up and pack or I will get George going. He is already zipping up the suitcase every time I get up to do something.

Right now I have him watching *Across the Universe*, a musical made from Beatles songs. I am enjoying it! Coo coo ka choo....

Earlier he watched Hannah Montana in concert. He seemed to enjoy it.

Tomorrow we start heading to La Porte, Indiana, where we will meet up with our friends Frankie and Dennis and see some of the areas where they bike and hang out.

Bicycle Friends are the Best!

September 26, 2017

It is Tuesday. We got up and got dressed. I concentrated on packing stuff into the containers and then showing George where to put the containers. It worked without me blowing a gasket.

We left Mackinaw City while it was still dark.

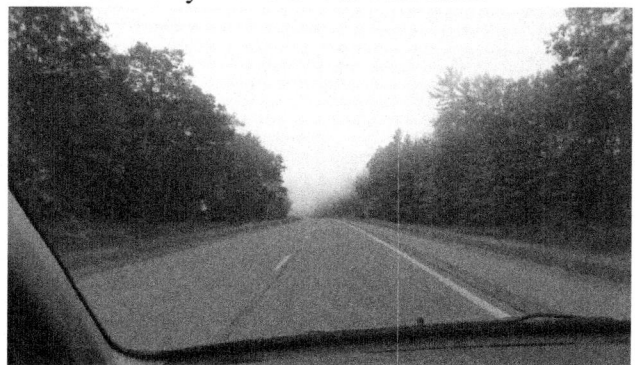

When we stopped at a wayside, I took George into the women's restroom after checking that it was empty. I changed his Depends and then I showed him to a bench in the shade.

"I have to go to the bathroom now. You stay here and I will be back in a bit," I tell him.

When I exit the bathroom, George is not on the bench. I panic a moment. I quickly walk around the restroom searching the area for George. Then I find him standing by the car on the passenger side, with his hand on the handle waiting for me to unlock it.

In the afternoon we stop at a grocery store. I park far from the building so we can exercise our legs. We walk back to the car in our usual formation... me in front, him following behind. When I get to the car, I unlock and get in. I look to the passenger side of the car. George is not there. I get out and scan the parking lot. No George.

I start walking back to the store when I spot him standing on the passenger side of a red van with his hand on the handle, looking around for me.

I had told our friends I would stay at a motel. I didn't want to impose too much. I stopped at a McDonald's to use the internet to hunt for motels by their home. I messaged Frankie to let her know we were 30 minutes away and she replied, "Just get your butts here! I am so excited."

That's what I love about Frankie!

She had a room ready and waiting for us. Dennis had just brought home groceries for our dinner.

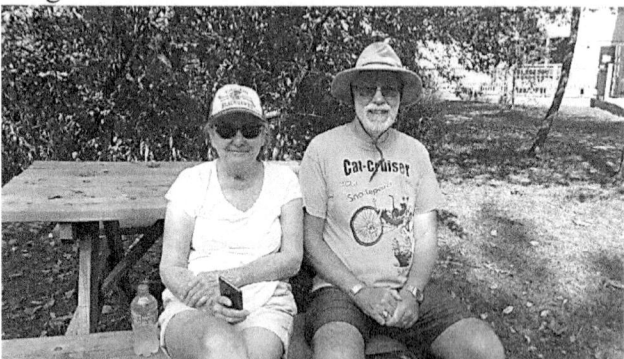

After relaxing in their backyard over a beer, we decided to go for a walk at the Dunes on Lake Michigan.

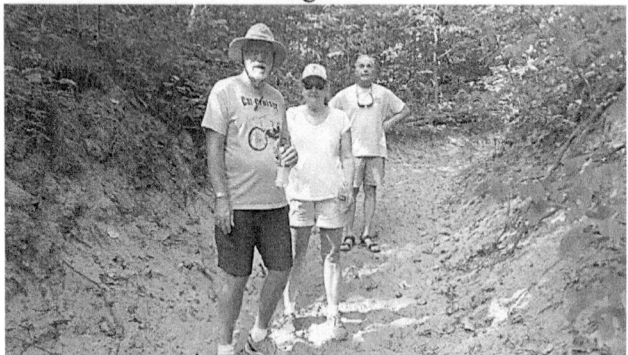

Climbing and walking on the sand was a challenge for George. I kept giving him my thumb to squeeze. Frankie took his other hand often.

It was warm. George and I both stepped into the water to cool off.

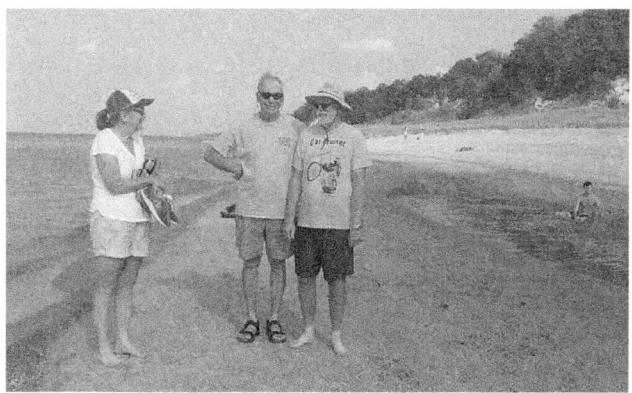

Dennis was hungry. (We call it "hangry." When you are so hungry you are anxious.) He had only had one half of a sandwich all day, he told us. We were moving very slowly with George in the loose sand. Frankie and I sent Dennis on ahead to get the car and meet us at the beach.

Dennis drove us to a restaurant for pizza. Dennis and Frankie insisted on paying the bill. When I protested Frankie said, "Let me looove you!"

Awww... I have no idea how to respond but to say, "THANK YOU!"

As Frankie says, "Bicycling friends are the best!"

Tomorrow the temperature is to drop 20 degrees and the wind may hit 20 mph. Of course, we plan on biking anyway!

Trike Ride in Indiana

September 27, 2017

George and I slept well at Frankie and Dennis's home in La Porte, Indiana. Frankie helped me make up a cushion on the floor for me to sleep. Since George jerks in his sleep I don't sleep well in a small bed with him, so the floor was perfect. Sometimes over the years I moved to the floor when we were home.

George only got up once during the night and the disposable mattress covers did their job, catching a small urine spill.

At breakfast, Frankie asked George how he was doing. "I got dementia," George told her.

"I know," Frankie said with concern. "How is that going for you?"

George shook his head and did his teary, silent laugh/cry.

Frankie took George's face in her hands and said, "You are a dear, sweet man, George. Everybody loves you." We all got teary.

Ahhh too deep, too emotional. I broke the spell. "It is what it is," I said. "That's what George would say, right George?"

He nods, and we talk about other things.

While they got their bikes packed in their van, I took pictures of the games that Frankie had given George last night.

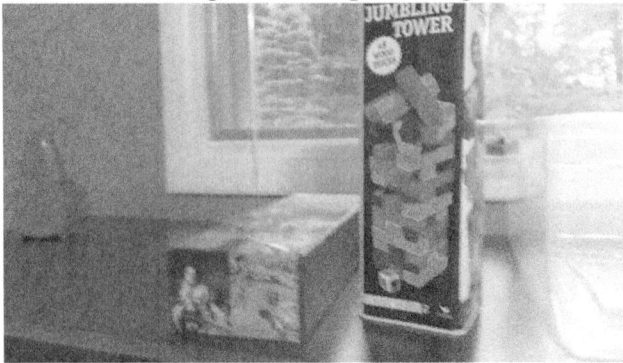

Frankie spent most of the time riding with George.

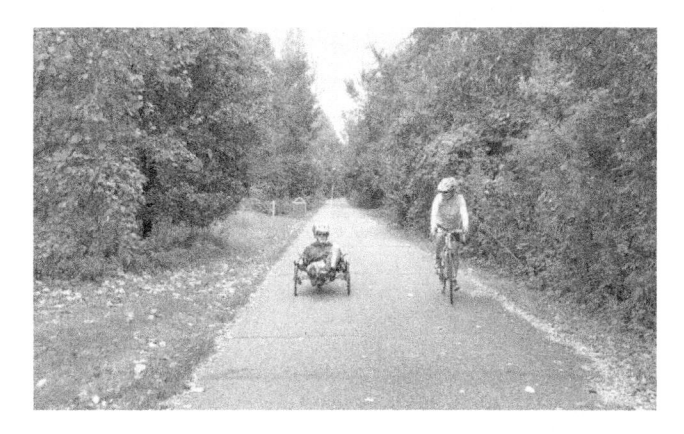

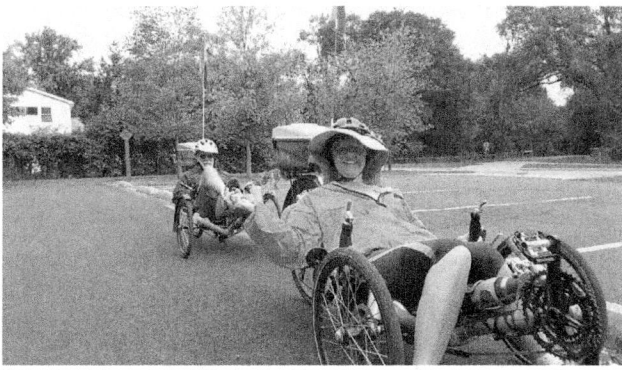

We rode about 15 miles and stopped at a park to use the restrooms (with flush toilets) and have a light snack.

On the way back Dennis stopped by a fence and said if you take a picture over this fence you will see a lawnmower graveyard.

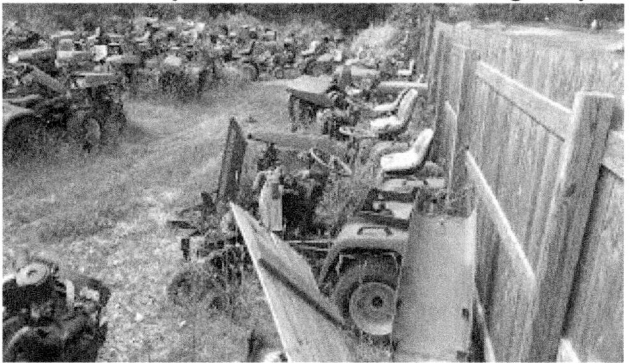

They all looked like John Deere mowers!

Back at home, Frankie and I called our friend Debra in Florida. We put her on speakerphone and had fun joking around with her. She was cooking dinner, and we could hear her chopping.

"Are you multi-tasking?" asked Frankie.

Frankie and Debra are both from the south and enjoyed a laugh over the fact that I didn't know what Frankie meant when she said that someone was "showing his ass."

To you northerners it means... misbehaving???

While I uploaded photos to this blog and checked email, Frankie watched TV with George. They watched *The Andy Griffith Show* and *M*A*S*H*.

After dinner I had to clean George. He stood still for me a long time while I wiped and washed and scrubbed and wiped some more. I am so lucky to have a cooperative "person." I worked up a sweat, and I swear we were in that bathroom 20 minutes.

I struggled for a moment about what to call him. I have heard the caregivers in our support group and in caregiver trainings call the care-receivers: "our person", "your person." That sounds respectful but cold. I am lucky to have a cooperative George.

I hadn't announced to my email list that I had launched a blog post and they didn't know how to find it without my email announcement. I was mistakenly not sending out an email every time I posted a blog entry to the list of friends and family because I thought I was "over-sharing." Everyone has their own lives and I didn't want to assume that mine was any more interesting than theirs. What I am hearing is that they want to follow our journey.

I have added the Dementia Divas to the email alert, and some have written they appreciate it and somehow it is helpful to them to read about our struggles and joys.

We have been gone a long time... the Wednesday before Irma hit Florida. I have had enough traveling for a while. I am ready to return home.

South

September 28, 2017

I woke but lay in bed hoping to get some extra sleep, knowing that driving home is the hard part of this trip. Today we start the drive home. Google maps say it is 1,117 miles to home.

Frankie gave George a cup of coffee and worked to distract him while I packed up. Then I enlisted George to help me carry things out to the car and showed him where to put each item. Yeah!!! Stress free packing!

We gave a big hug to our friends and promised to party when they come to Florida this winter.

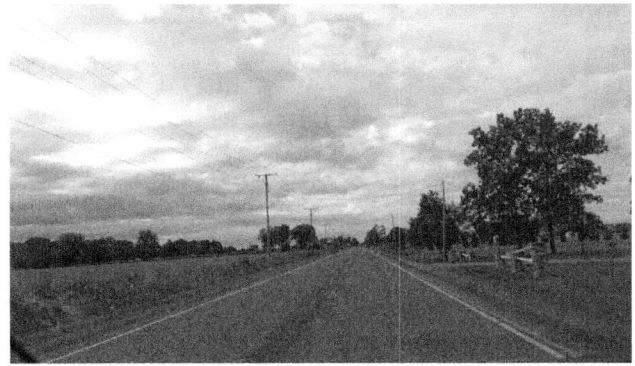

Dennis provided instructions to take 421, which was a good plan. I loved 421. There was light traffic and the road was heading straight and directly *south*.

Straight through the grain belt with golden fields and huge combines.

We got onto interstate 65. Wow, what a big difference: faster; congestion; huge trucks; construction.

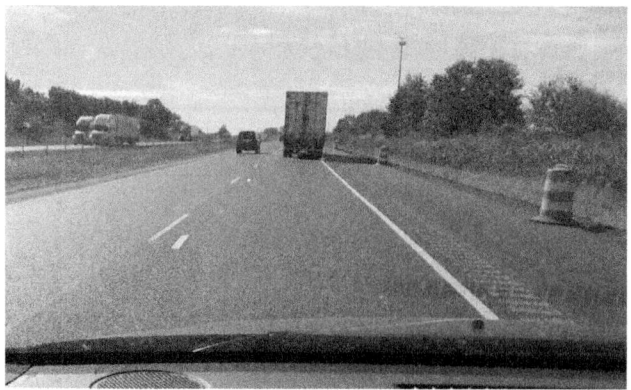

We went for walks at waysides. If George ever wanders and I have to call the police, I will tell them to check red vans. George might be sitting in the passenger side or hanging onto the passenger door handle waiting for me.

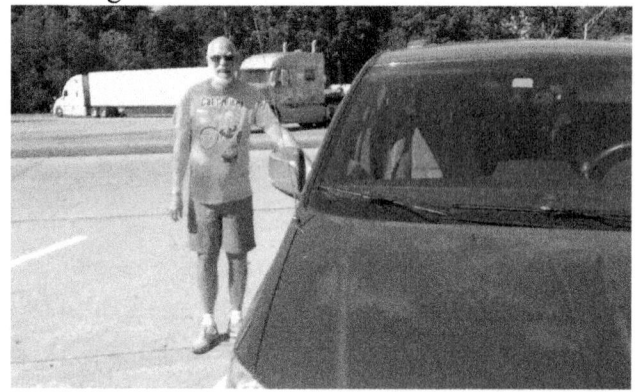

I can see why people do fast food. We went to a grocery store and got salad and soup and then had difficulty finding a park with a picnic table and bathrooms.

There were no bathrooms in the park. I headed back into town to go to the CVS.

When we got to CVS, I started walking toward the entrance and turned around to make sure George was walking behind me.

He was walking behind me but he had wet shorts from overflowing his depends. I put off going to CVS and found a sports park nearby using the GPS.

Fortunately, there was no game going on, so the place was empty, but the restrooms were open and had water. Clean, clean, clean - then back to CVS for more wipes and a snack.

Drive, drive, drive. We enter the hills of Kentucky and I get tired.

We stop at a wayside and get a coupon book. We walk around. I pick out a motel for $59/night.

It is not by the Interstate, it is through town four miles. I am hungry and tired, and when we pull in I am disappointed. I wanted a nice place with crisp sheets and a good breakfast and a roomy bathroom.

We stand outside the car and I debate. The neighborhood isn't the greatest. A guest pulls in with their radio thumping loudly. I decide to choose a different motel.

I go back to the highway. There is a bunch all along one street near the highway. So I pull into one. "We will check on the price of this one, and if it is too much we will go to the next one until we find something that fits us," I say to George.

But I am not a good bargain hunter. I am tired and hungry, and I smell pooh, and I just want a nice clean place where I can do laundry and relax.

The first place was $107 for one night. I took it.

I clean his bottom and we walk over to Wendy's fast food place. I get us each a baked potato with cheese and broccoli and a salad without the chicken.

In our room after dinner, George follows me closely. When I say closely, I mean that when I stand at the sink rinsing out a rag, he is there with his belly touching my elbow. Sometimes I have to gently put him back a couple steps so I can move around.

I have him go with me to the laundry room to put a load in the washer. He stands next to me right in front of the washer, taking half my working space.

Back in our room, I clean him up again and take him in the shower. Naked, I help him dry, get him dressed, and set him in front of a TV show. Then I jump in the shower myself....

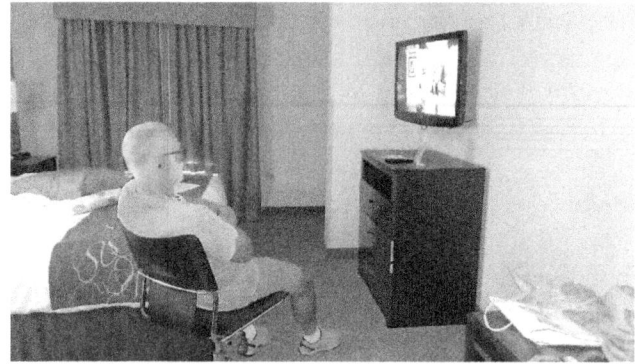

I read my email and discover my friend Connie was cleaning up tree debris after the hurricane and fell down some steps and broke both ankles. "OH NO!!"

She cares for her husband, Jerry, who has gone blind with macular degeneration. Jerry is able to stay at home by himself and care for his dogs. But he relies on Connie to help him get places and so much more.

Now she is in the hospital with all kinds of metal contraptions keeping one ankle together. Her other ankle will need a boot. Her daughter is already there to help.

How quickly a caregiver can become incapacitated. I need to have a plan. When I get home I plan to investigate the memory care places. I know our friends Debra and Glen could probably watch George a day or two until George's daughter could get here or until he could be placed in a memory care facility.

We need to prepare for surprises.

Zoo Stop and a Mishap

September 29, 2017

Are we tired of driving and riding still? YES WE ARE!

The interstate is moving, but crowded and stressful. I want to get off!!!!

George, for someone with Alzheimer's or Dementia, is riding very, very well. He is quiet and still.

He never complains (he can no longer formulate the sentences to do that). He never whines.

Last night we stayed at a nice motel. I wanted to take advantage of it. After a nice breakfast in their lobby, I took George into the fitness room. It has been a while since I have taken him to a gym... maybe three months. He didn't even try to do the weights.

He climbed onto the treadmill. I got it going for him real, real slow. He was hanging on but taking smaller and smaller steps. His feet were almost off the back and he was bent over walking the treadmill. I kept pushing his butt to get him to stand up better. After about two minutes at the most, we gave up.

I was able to do some weights and do about 15 minutes on the treadmill while George stood watching the TV.

Back in our room I set him up in front of cartoons and I packed up the bags. Thank you, George, for watching TV!

I was so tired of driving the interstate. It is so impersonal, so fast; the scenery is mostly the same wide path through the woods with construction cones.

I saw an exit for US 41 and thought I might try that.

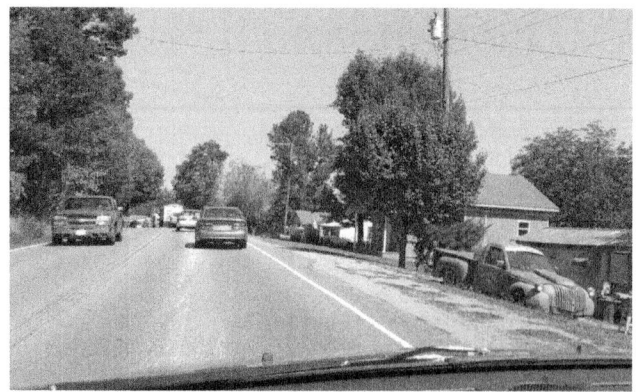

It was nice for a while, but then it was cities and stop-lights. I got back on Hwy 24.

A billboard advertising the zoo did the trick on me and lured me into Chattanooga.

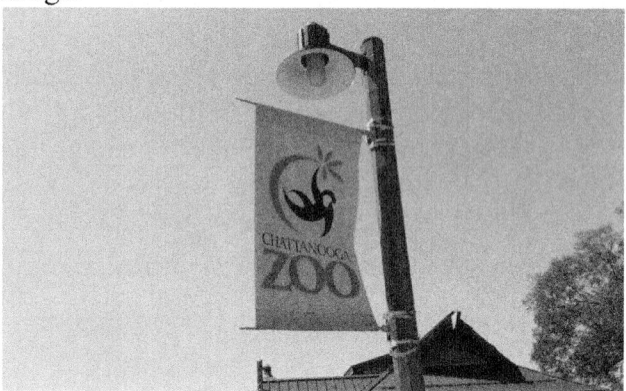

Shortly after we entered the zoo, I lost George. I made a video and put it up on YouTube. Go to http://bit.ly/GeorgeZoo. You won't want to miss this story. While you are there hit the thumbs up and the subscribe button. Thank you!

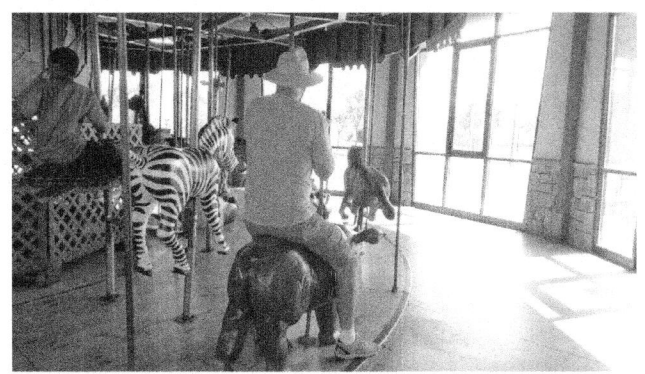

After that incident I saw how much like a little boy he has become.

At one point I stopped to look closer at an animal, and George got caught up following a woman and her children. I wondered if it freaked her out to have this stumbling, smiling old guy following her children around.

I called him back to me.

Later, I pulled off Interstate 75 and used the GPS to find a Mexican restaurant. It took me down a road into a community with a lot of Hispanic businesses.

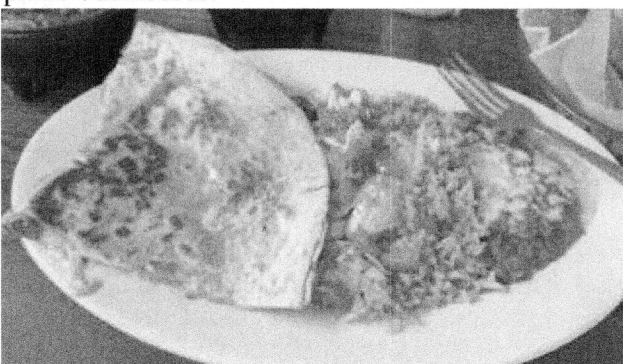

The restaurant TV was reporting on Puerto Rico's disaster and the recovery efforts there and in Mexico City after the earthquake.

It puts our journey in perspective.

After going through Atlanta I began searching for a motel. We went to four motels before settling down on the fifth.

The first didn't have a handicap shower or tub with a bar to grab available.

The second was closed and under construction.

The third I got out of the car and approached the lobby. I saw the couch in the lobby was dark on the upper back and on the arms from the dirt of thousands of hands. As I turned and said, "Oh no, we aren't staying here!" a man came out smelling like whiskey.

The fourth was in the same neighborhood with litter-strewn streets.

It took over an hour to get just a few blocks between all these hotels.

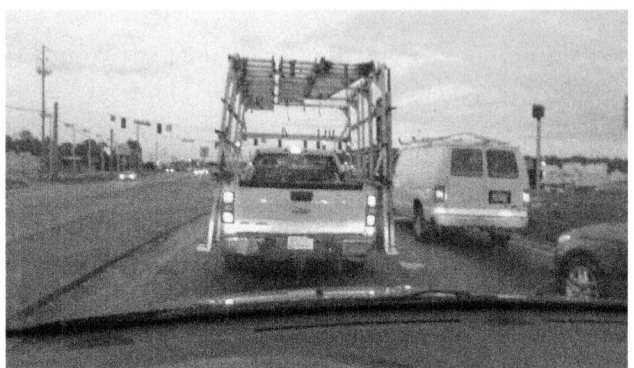

Finally we found a place in a better neighborhood and clean enough with a handicap shower. We were too tired to use the shower tonight.

George is sleeping as I finish off this post.

I tried to get him to scooch down in the bed. His head was bent sideways against the headboard; he was leaning funny. He could not comprehend what I was saying or gesturing. He is worn out.

I think we have about 400 miles to home.

Back Home

September 30, 2017

Thanks for checking in on us.

We made it home OK around 7 p.m., both of us tired and not wanting to look at the inside the car for a while.

I will write more later... when the energy returns.

****

I didn't sleep well last night. I cried a few tears as I remembered George at the zoo on the merry-go-round. (If you didn't watch the video it is at: http://bit.ly/GeorgeZoo)

Driving... in high-speed close traffic and in close proximity to lots of big trucks can cause insomnia due to increased adrenaline secretions... that's my theory.

I tried to sleep late, but my inner clock knows when it is daytime. We are up around 6 a.m.

Our last day on the road I pulled off at High Falls State Park. We needed a walk and to commune with nature.

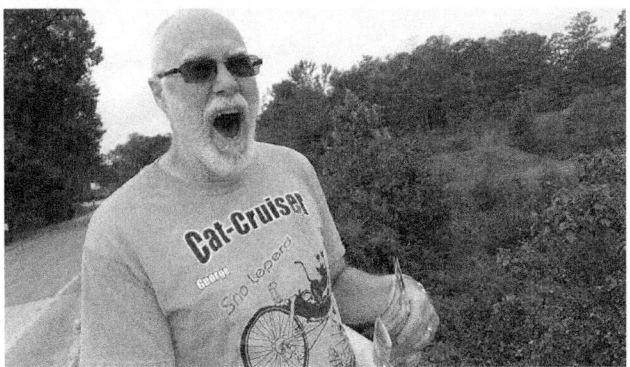

We each carry our coffees. When I put mine down to take a picture, George puts his down. When I take a sip, George takes a sip.

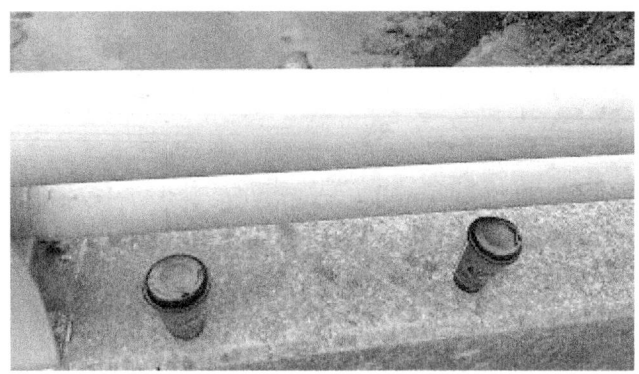

When we got to the trail, it was mostly rocks and stairs going down. We only got halfway down when I realized this was not a good idea with George at his stage of dementia. His balance and strength are not what they were just a few months ago.

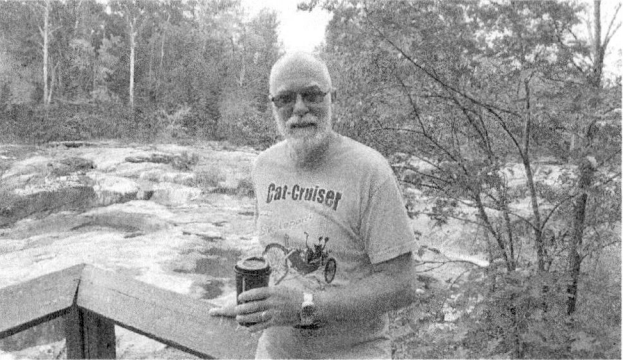

I make the decision to not go any further.

The other day we were climbing stairs in a motel and I remembered just three years ago we would race and George would win. He could bounce up those steps.

As I drive I keep stopping to try something else to give me energy again.

Finally we cross the border! We get grapefruit juice samples to drink at the wayside. I use the internet there to find a carwash further down the road.

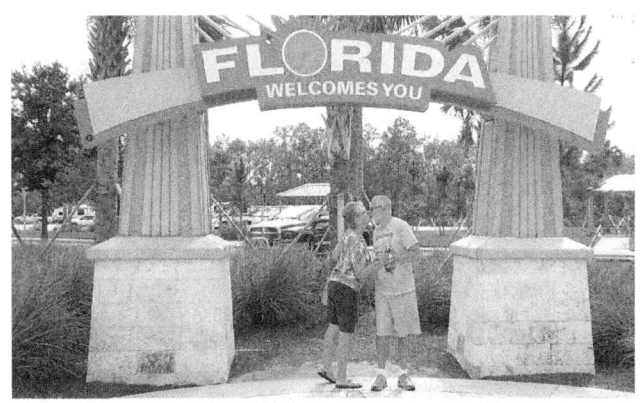

It is pouring rain when I pull into the car wash. But our car is so filthy with bugs and dirt and brake dust on the wheels that I drive in anyway.

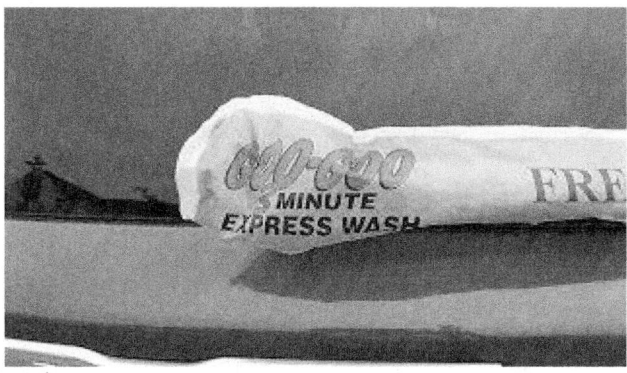

I feel clean!

When we get to Gainesville, I have visions of spending the night. I am so tired that we just might order food in.

It takes me a good ten minutes or longer to go three blocks with several stops at each light. Traffic is terrific. It is 5 p.m. on a Friday night.

I finally get to the motel I have selected from the coupon book and I learn that this is a Gator game weekend. Rooms don't go for less than $150 per night.

We walked from the motel to the end of the street and I did some leg kicks, knee lifts, punches and squats trying to get my blood moving and build up to going back to sit in that car for more hours.

It works. I am feeling up to doing it. We get back on the interstate and pass Paynes Prairie which is full of water from the flooding after Irma. The traffic is zipping; I am feeling good.

Then it starts to pour again and the traffic slows to a crawl. Sigh

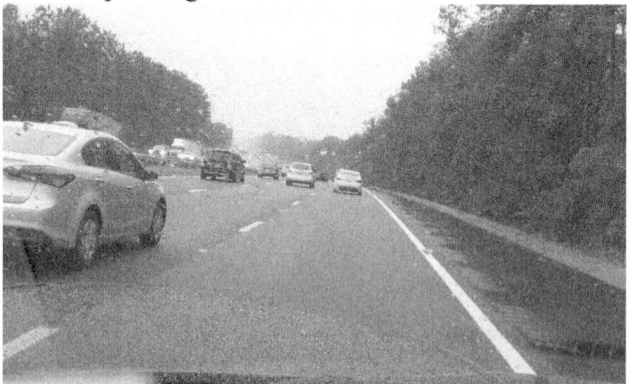

I turn off the Interstate early. I am hoping to find a restaurant and grocery store too. Our friends Debra and Margaret emptied our fridge after the storm knocked out the power for several days. THANK YOU dear friends!

We turn onto our street and there is our home... it looks so different without the big shade tree.

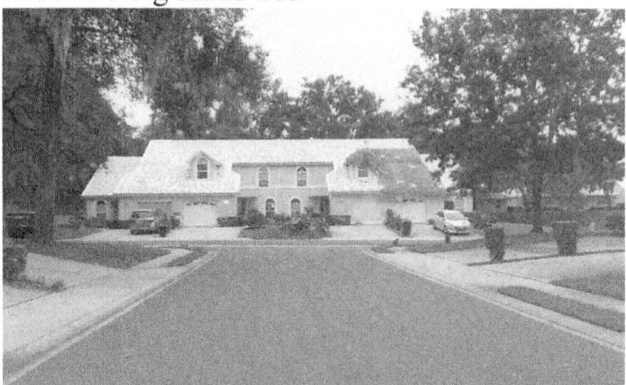

I just bring a few things in and then we walk over to Margaret and Zip's to get our mail. I had asked them to take in our mail for a very short period of time during our escape from Irma. It turned out to be almost a whole month!

Back at home, George watched a nature film while I did a little unpacking.

One of our renters, Tirso, came home and greeted us. He had fled the storm and was unable to find gasoline until he turned onto Hwy 10 in northern Florida. He left one day after us.

George finished out his evening coloring while I sat with him checking email and uploading pictures to this blog.

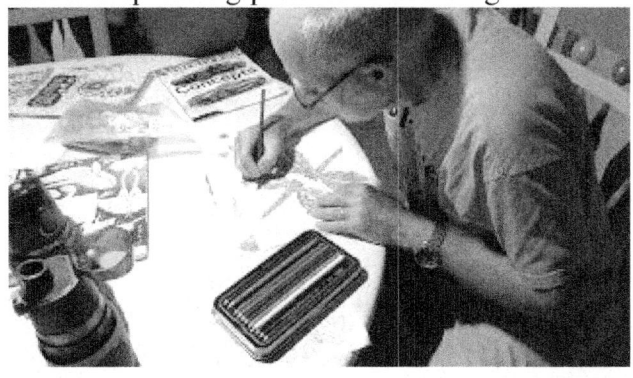

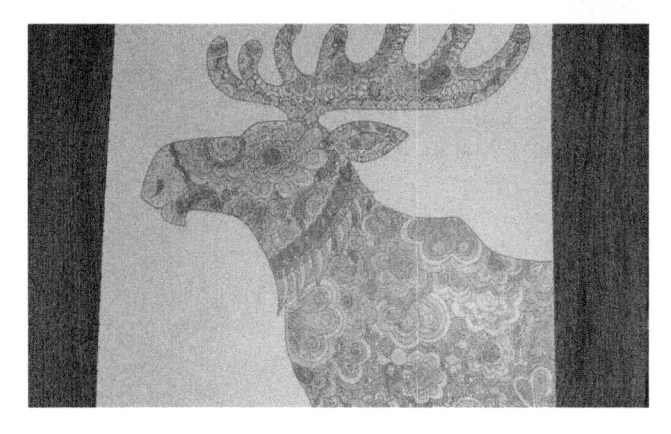

Caregiver: Entertainment Engineer, Snot Cop

October 18, 2017

    This week the Dementia Divas and Princes asked me about the specifics. They want to be ready when their time to deal with incontinence arrives. It will come if your loved one lives long enough. I was going to include instructions and tips here in this post. But I have decided to create a separate post entitled Dementia Doodoo Diva. What do you think?

    In this post, I will talk about keeping George active and trying to satisfy his "go and do" urge. This "go and do" need is something that is not uncommon among persons with dementia.

    In our support group there are persons with dementia who want to go and do and there are persons with dementia who don't want to go anywhere or do anything. I am lucky that George wants to go and do. Though sometimes it drives me nuts that he just can't sit and do nothing at times, I would much rather he wanted to go so that I could go.

    Since we returned from our Hurricane Irma escape trip we have biked and walked and visited folks and gone to meetings and parks.

    We continue to ride bike. George seems to still enjoy it. He gets the bikes out and is anxious to go. Folks who know George from his days at the Floral City bike shop or on the trail chatting with folks will yell out, "Hi George!" as they pass. He waves at everyone.

    When we ride, he keeps up sometimes, and sometimes he lags behind and I have to turn around or stop to wait for him. Many Tuesdays and Thursdays for half the ride, our friend Zip rides with George so I can enjoy the ride without having to watch my rearview mirror.

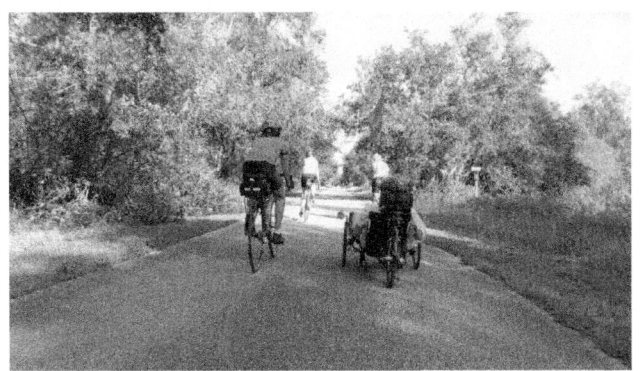

Often, George doesn't shift gears on the trike to prepare to stop or climb a hill. I asked at the bike shop about an automatic shifter.... They can't put one on his current trike. So I would have to buy a new one. $7,000 for the trike and shift package! Oh my! I guess I will just keep trying to help him shift at the intersections. Or maybe I will send him to adult day care once in a while so I can ride longer and faster. It will take a lot of day care to use up $7,000!

The worry is that crossing intersections he can be very, very sloooow. I and others are telling him, "Pedal, George, pedal!" But he is usually in the wrong gear and pedals verrrry slooooow. I tell myself that if he gets hit, it's a better way to go than this slow fade he is living through. But of course it would be tragic and it might not kill him, just hurt him. That isn't good either. And that isn't even considering the poor soul driving the car that hits him.

So if anyone out there knows of a cheaper solution to the shifting problem, let me know. I thought about a tandem trike. Those are way too expensive also.

****

Though we came out without damage to our home from Hurricane Irma, our nextdoor neighbors had a tree land on their roof causing the tiles to break.

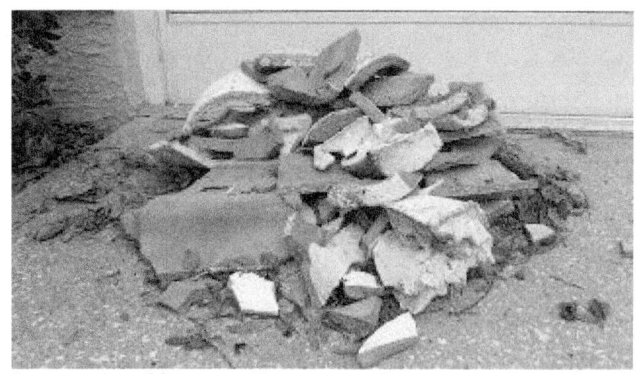

Before they arrived home, George and I scooped up the debris.

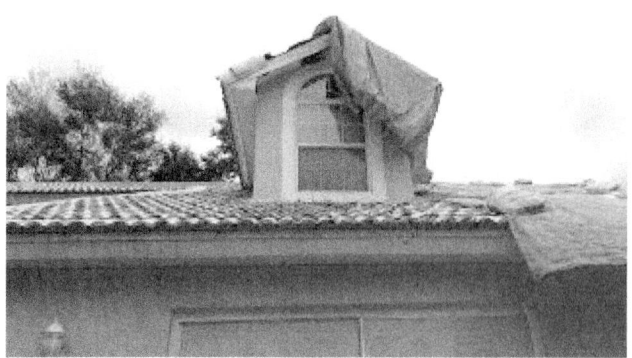

Respite

On Tuesday and Thursday afternoons I have a woman coming in to provide respite care. Her name is Jean. Jean is pleasant and positive and we like her.

Jean isn't as fit as George and so when she takes him for a walk she thinks going around the block is a long way.

Next time she comes I am going to give her better instructions on how to deal with George's toileting. The last two times I got home from my time away George had pooh in his disposable diaper/pants.

She asks him if he wants help and he refuses. I will instruct her in how to do it in a take-charge matter-of-fact way. "Let's go into the bathroom and clean you up."

What do I do with my respite time? I often feel I need to get as much into and out of these hours as I can. So I feel a little pressure to use that time wisely.

The fall has been *very* hot. During respite time I have to find indoor places to hang out away from the heat.

Often times I have taken my computer over to the neighborhood clubhouse. I spent $400 on a course to get re-certified as a fitness instructor, personal trainer and senior fitness specialist. But so far I haven't gotten through much of the training materials. Sometimes I do that during respite or while George is watching movies. It isn't so much time chunks as it is priorities and energy and drive.

Some of my fellow Dementia Divas stay home while their relief help is in the house. I do my banking online at home but then I want to get away so I don't hear them. I am always listening for his movements and his needs. I want to be able to shut down that part of my brain for a little while.

Activities for me during respite include:
- Socializing with friends
- Time in the gym lifting weights
- Walking (though in the heat that isn't an option)
- Blogging
- Catching up on calls and emails and paperwork
- Getting my hair cut or nails done
- Shopping.

Activities for George:
- Movies
- Going places (with me)
- Eating
- 24-piece puzzles
- Coloring
- Sorting different colored poker chips, cards, things
- Sorting coins
- Building wooden block towers

- Walking (with me or Jean)
- Yoga (with me)
- Exercises (with me)
- Visiting others who are homebound (with me).

We just went to a social gathering and there was food out. I handed George the pistachios and he was content to shell them and eat them. I didn't think about that. Maybe I can buy a big bag and have him shell nuts. It is also an activity for him while everyone else is chatting. He wasn't grabbing so much to eat when he had the nuts to shell. Cool!

The other day when I picked him up from day care he was working with one of those plastic kindergarten toys. It has oversized screws and nuts of different sizes and colors. He was putting the nuts onto the bolts.

Jodie tried to interest him in one of those boards with different latches and locks. It didn't seem to keep his interest long. But maybe we can watch the thrift shop for toy tools that work.

Someone suggested stringing Cheerios for the birds. I got the Cheerios, and then we ate them. I never got the string and big needle. The problem with that activity is that I would have to do it with him.

He used to play games on his iPad. But now, even easy games have things that pop up that get him off in other places on the internet.

This week he turned 70. He got a lot of wonderful greetings on Facebook. Since he never looks on Facebook, it was time for me to end his account. They only offer the option to delete it if he is dead. So I said he was dead.

Going Bonkers

I think I am going a bit crazy. I mean I would never have spent money before on getting my nails done. The manicure is another sign I am going a bit toward the nutty side of the sliding scale. But my nails were breaking easy and with all the rag squeezing and butt cleaning I didn't want to deal with breaking nails and such.

Which reminds me, I removed my wedding ring the other day. While squeezing a rag the ring gouged skin off a knuckle yet again. Enough! I don't want open wounds on my hands with the stuff I get into.

Another sign I am not acting logically... today I signed us up for a fundraising walk for an organization that helps caregivers by giving them small grants to pay for respite care. The fundraising walk cost us $50, almost the cost of a full day of day care.

The other day I sat eating cookies while reading instructions from my doctor on how to lose weight.

I don't mind being a bit off-center. It gives me permission to do stuff differently... maybe with a bit more pizazz.

I was commiserating with a fellow Dementia Diva about worrying about the money lasting until we women die. Then I told her my sister said, "Don't worry, it is only money," and "It will all work out just fine."

I said, "Well, maybe I will get dementia and money won't matter to me anymore."

She responded: "You are my sunshine - such a kick! So the light at the end of the tunnel could be the darn train!!"

It is great to have these fellow caretakers sharing their journey with us.

The folks with dementia too are sharing their experiences. Herb Terry had an article on the front page of the *Citrus County Chronicle* (local newspaper) about his experience with dementia. It really hit me how very aware he is of what is happening to him.

George isn't very verbal, so the only clue we have that he is aware is his teary laugh and his self-introduction, "I have dementia."

More Happenings

A couple weeks after our return from our Hurricane Irma escape the piles of brush from the downed trees and limbs were removed from the sides of the road.

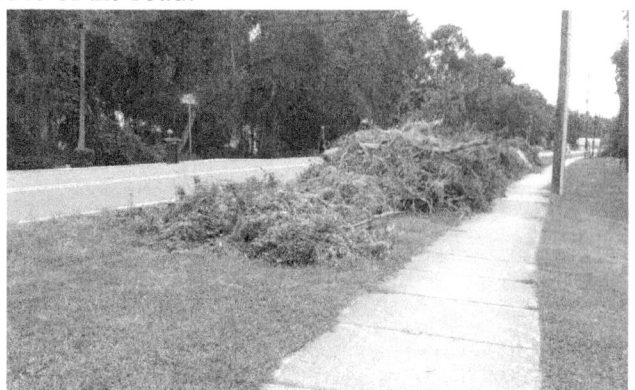

I drive us closer to Cooter pond to walk around it. We used to walk the three miles round trip from home, but now that is too far for George without lots of long bench sits... which drive him nuts..."Ready to go?" he says over and over.

Our friend Regis had given George a coloring book of hot cars. George seems to enjoy coloring them which keeps him occupied while I cook or make calls. He says, "See?" And then, "See?" And then, "See?" And each time, I try to come up with an original comment in return.

"Wow, look at that!" I say. "What kind of car is that?" I ask. "Is that my car?"

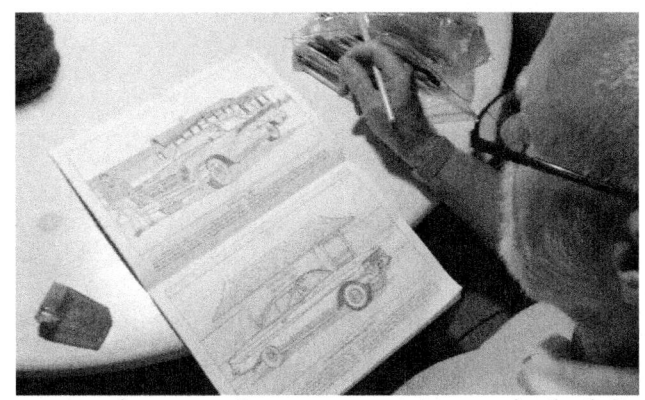

After returning from our Irma escape trip, we looked forward to breakfasts with our bike group. They greeted us warmly. We are so blessed with their ongoing acceptance and inclusion. One of the hazards for caregivers and those with dementia is social isolation. Not for us! Thanks to George's smiles and quiet, cooperative demeanor and their love. Thank you!

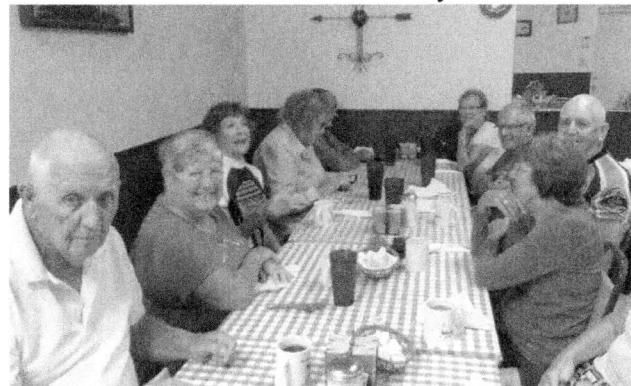

On a trike ride south on the trail we stopped at Townsen Park to see how high the water had risen. It was interesting; Hurricane Irma came through weeks ago and yet the river just peaked a few days ago in this area and will peak a few days after this picture further downstream. Some people in neighborhoods along the river are still wading and boating to reach their homes.

I was glad to see that our favorite tree in Townsen Park was still standing, and there is an old oak nearby that survived the storm also.

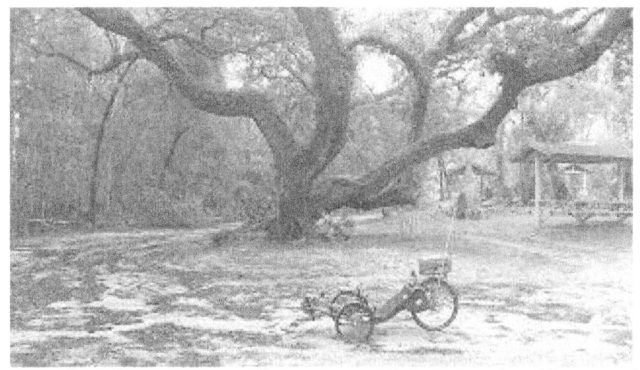

On our way back to town, George and I turned off onto the ramp that would take us up to 44 and the sidewalk to Winn Dixie. The ramp had not been cleared yet. I stopped and tried to pull things off the trail, but all I did was gain an appreciation for the volunteers and staff who did all the work to clear branches entangled with vines all along the trail and roads in Citrus County.

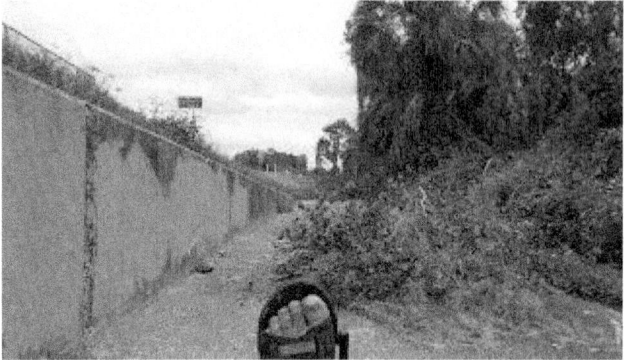

On Sunday the drum circle was going on at Fort Island Beach (on the Gulf near Crystal River). I picked up our friend Jerry who loves these things and we went to do a little drumming and dancing on the beach. You may remember me mentioning his wife, Connie, who broke both her ankles while cleaning up after Irma.

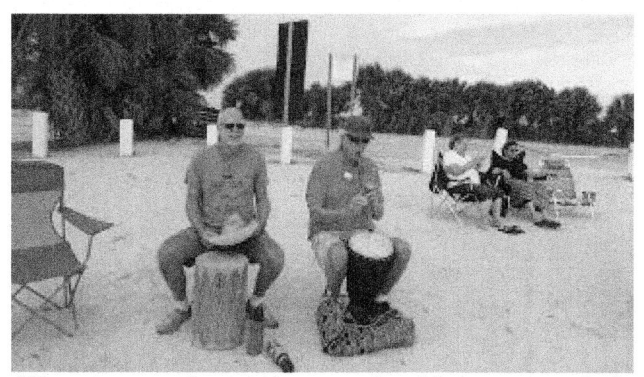

George likes to watch movies on the big screen. I don't have headphones that work with our big dumb TV. The noise makes it hard for me to concentrate on tasks I want to attend to. So sometimes I bring George into the den with me and use the headphones with his iPad. Nice and quiet. At least until his movie ends... or messes up... or loses his attention.

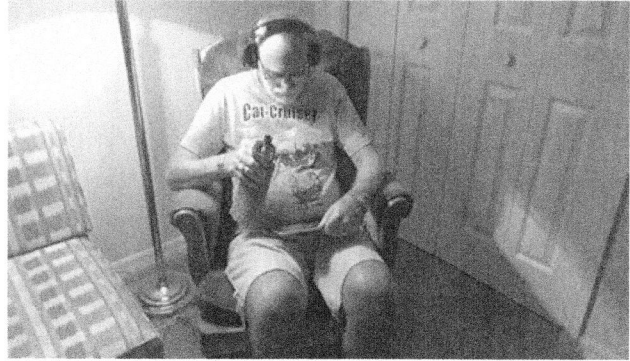

One of the people renting a bedroom from us got sick and had to return to her parents' home. The day she moved her things out she left me a beautiful bouquet of flowers and a thank you card. Thank you, Lydia!

I decided to leave that bedroom open for a few months because I want it available for family and friends who are coming to visit this fall and winter. George's daughter is coming to visit for a couple weeks so she can assist me in caring for George. I am looking forward to having some time to sort through some stuff and clean and organize the garage and attic and closets.

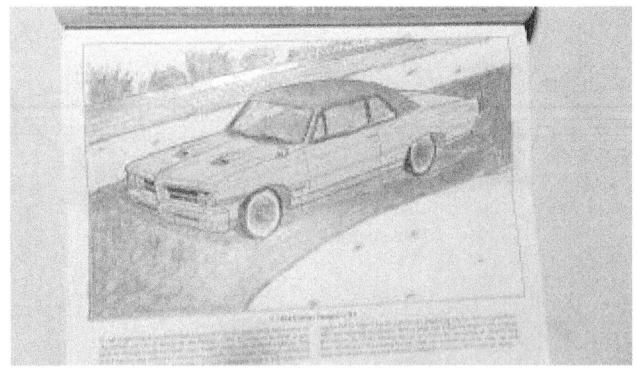

Debra and Glen drove us to The Villages for dinner and dancing on the square. While we were at The Villages and I was up dancing without George, I had to keep one eye on George. He got up a couple times and started walking away, attracted by the vendor booths around the square. I took him for a stroll then around to see the vendors. I thought it would satisfy him. One of the vendors was selling belts and George had just outgrown his belt. I got him a new one that should grow and shrink with him. He has grown from a 28 waist to a 34 waist. As he grows I put his old shorts in a pile in his closet. He will someday not eat so well and his waistline will shrink again.

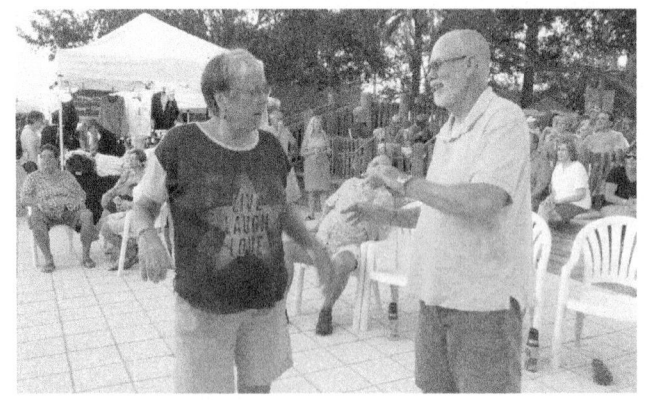

Snot Cop

I have become the snot cop. Watching for the dribble and the dangle so I can remind him to blow his nose or catch it with something myself. This is another milestone that I have to wrap my mind and heart around. My old man with a snot dangle - oh my. Poor George is losing more and more of the man he was.

He usually dribbles in the morning at breakfast. I am thinking I will get tissues and keep them close to the dining table.

He used to have a very distinct sound when he blew his nose. If I lost him in a store or a crowd it wasn't for long. He would blow his nose and I knew which way to go find him. Now his blow is quiet.

Sometimes during the day I have to remind him to blow his nose. If he is real foggy I hold the hanky to his nose and tell him to blow... no horn blow now.

Poop Police

My sense of smell is playing tricks on me. I can't trust my nose anymore. I smell pooh so I check and there is nothing. I don't smell pooh and do a periodic check anyway and there is pooh.

Even so, I guess among the Dementia Divas and Princes, I am looked to for information. Probably because of this blog I am now looked at as the one with experience and expertise on how to deal with incontinence. I am still learning. My method works on George; it might not work on anyone else. Each person with dementia travels a different journey with different behaviors, abilities, and emotions. Each caregiver comes to the task with different talents, abilities, and issues of their own.

The trajectory for Alzheimer's puts bowel incontinence closer to the end stage. George isn't near the end stage yet.

George's brain damage has occurred so that he doesn't sense he has a back body anymore. It is evident when he showers and only the front of his body that he can see gets washed and dried if I don't assist him.

Rarely does he go to the toilet to pooh, though it does happen on rare occasions. He goes pee in the toilet about 1/3 of the time.

I have wondered if he has no sense of his anus and backside, then he could poop while I am cleaning him. Well, since that thought occurred, it has happened. I am wiping and wiping and not getting to the end. It is like a magician pulling all this stuff out of a hat. I keep scooping. I keep telling George, "Hold still, I am not done yet... not yet, there is more to clean."

This week I finished cleaning his bottom and put him in the shower while I got undressed to join him. I step into the shower and see him standing with his hand full of pooh and more on the floor of the shower. He is totally unaware of what is happening; he was just trying to rinse the stuff off his hands.

"Whoops! Stay, don't move," I said, and stepped back out of the shower and got some wipes and the waste basket to clean up. As I clean him I try to comfort him: "This is just the journey we are on." If he is aware at that moment, he needs comforting. If he is aware he won't be aware for long. That thought comforts me.

I now have him face his sink while I clean his bottom. I have to remind him not to move. "Not yet, I am not done yet." The other day, while I was cleaning his bottom, he picked up his toothbrush and toothpaste and brushed his teeth. Ha-ha.

I have a couple objects I toss into his sink and tell him to play with them. But they don't keep his interest. Maybe I should get some of those oversized plastic bolts and nuts....

So, anyway - I am going to do a separate post dedicated to toileting. I hope it either helps other caregivers or at least provides someone a laugh or a giggle or a smile.

Dementia DooDoo Diva

Alzheimer's is Crappy

October 31, 2017

Warning, this post is full of specifics about dealing with incontinence. It is focusing on stuff I have learned while taking care of the incontinence issues. A Dementia Diva asked me for details since many/most caregivers may be washing bottoms now or later.

So for those of you who are just checking in on George and I and our lives, you may want to skip this post. It's pretty shitty.

Respect

You don't know at any moment how much your loved one comprehends or understands. So always treat them with respect. If you are tired or frustrated try hard to think how they must feel if they are having a cognitive moment and you have to wipe their bottom.

If I notice George is doing his nervous laugh, I say, "It is what it is, George." Or I say, "Dang dementia, that part of the brain just disappeared. That's OK; we will just deal with it."

The pictures below are from a display at the Floral City Library put together by Ed Youngblood for the Alzheimer's Family Organization fundraising walk in October 2017.

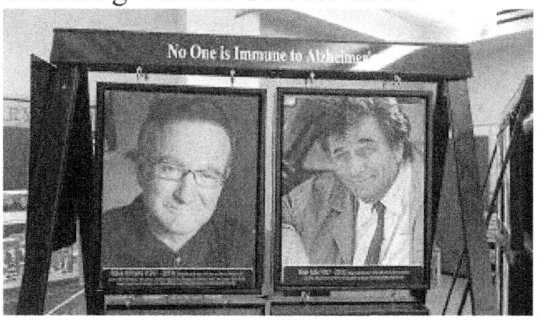

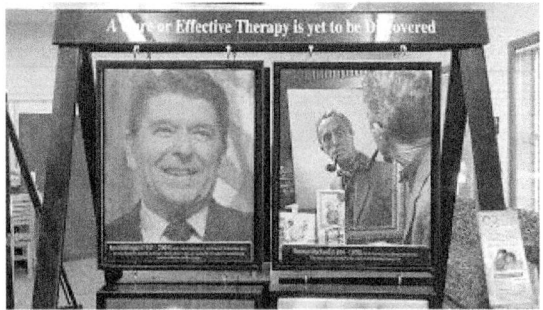

These people all had dementia. If they survived long enough, they had to have their bottoms wiped by someone else.

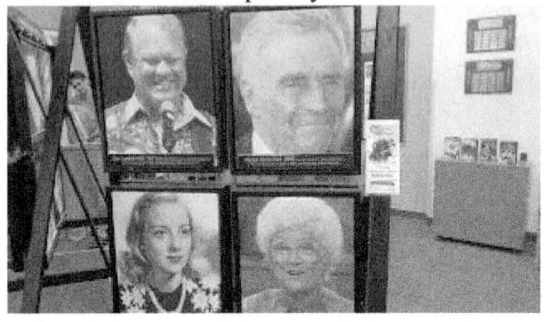

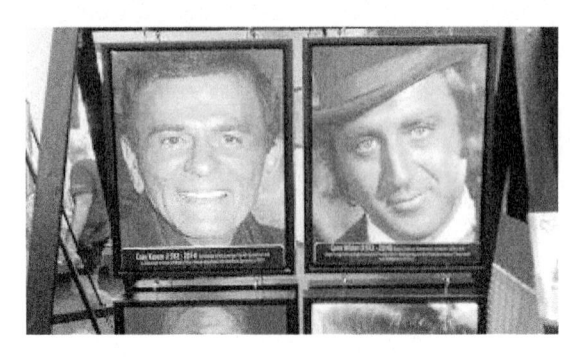

Things That I Have Tried

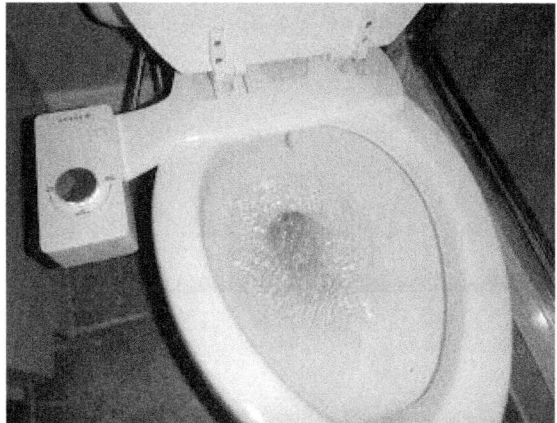

I tried the Tushy bidet that you attach to your toilet. It works well for me, but for a hairy bottom that has been sitting on the stuff, it doesn't have a wide enough or strong enough spray. So I stopped using it on George.

I tried using wash rags instead of disposable wipes. It requires *lots* of water rinses and sometimes washing out the rag in the toilet and I *really* don't like using my sink where I brush my teeth and wash my face to rinse out the rag. I still use the rag sometimes and I carry one in the "diaper bags."

Transition to Diapers

The transition to wearing diapers or urinary pads may be the hardest part for your loved one. Here is how it went for us. First with urinary incontinence, and then with bowel incontinence it was a one-two-three-strikes-you're-out process.

A friend had brought some urinary incontinence pads over for us to try after seeing George with wet pants.

When he had another accident, I mentioned he might want to start with the pad ... he refused. He had another accident after I had asked if he needed to use the restroom and he refused to use the restroom. So I talked with him and said this was just part of the journey we were on and he was going to have to start wearing the pad eventually. I offered it; he refused.

The third time I put the pad in his pants and said, "Just try them and see. If after a week the pad doesn't get wet, you can try going without it again." That worked.

When the third time with bowel incontinence occurred I took all his underwear out of his drawer and placed the full Depends pants on the back of the toilet.

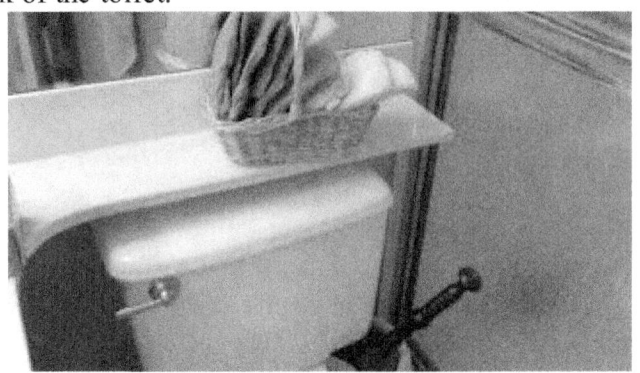

Checking For Pooh

A Diva asked how often I check him. If I don't smell anything I still check him three times a day. More if I suspect a bulge, smell, or stain.

After our morning walk or yoga we walk right into the bathroom to check. I say, "Let's go right into the bathroom and clean up." If he doesn't follow it might be because he didn't understand. Since sometimes those with dementia only understand a few words at a time I shorten the instructions. "Bathroom; Follow me; Clean up."

Before we go somewhere I may say, "Let's get you cleaned up before we go."

I have learned that I need to not just peek in the front and back, but I need to pull the Depends down to his knees to check. Sometimes the urine settles toward the bottom and there is no evidence at the top. And if you don't catch that, an hour later he might be walking in public with wet pants or getting your furniture wet (or someone else's ... argh!)

The other day I smelled old pooh. I checked him twice that afternoon. Nothing. Later I found he had one walnut-sized pooh stuck in his crack. It didn't stain the diaper so I didn't see it when I checked his pants. Now if I smell something, I use a wet-wipe to see if there is anything hiding.

Later I will go through a typical step-by-step process of cleaning him.

Incontinence Supplies

I used to be careful not to buy disposable stuff. Reuse, Reduce, Recycle was my mantra. Now I love disposables. I tell myself it is only temporary.

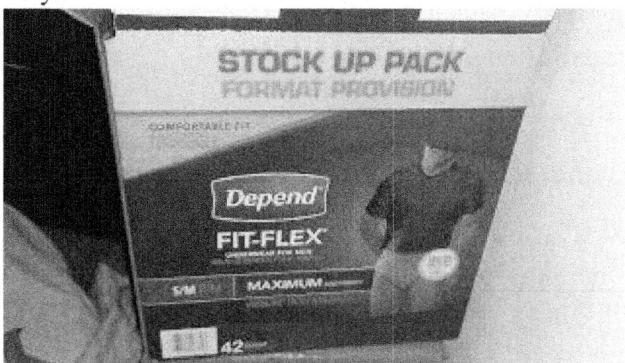

Maximum Absorbency Depends Brand - I get them in large quantities from Amazon. They were 50 cents each but last time I ordered them they were up to $.59 each. (After this post I learned that if your loved one is a U.S. Veteran they can get incontinence products for free through the VA. Speak to their VA doctor.)

I keep the boxes in George's closet which is right outside the master bath. I keep a basket on the back of the toilet with a few Depends in it. If I keep the number small I can notice when he has been changing them himself at night.

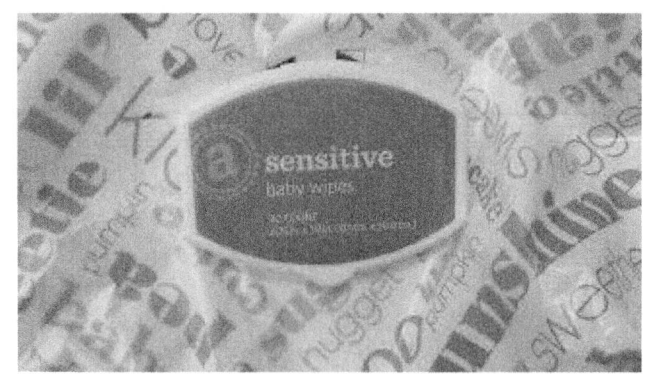

Sensitive Baby Wipes distributed by Amazon. So far these are the biggest and best. I can wet them and soap them and scrub and they don't fall apart. Do not flush any wet wipes. They are bad for the sewer system.

Plastic Shopping Bags

We don't use cloth bags at the store now, these plastic bags are very handy waste containers. They line a small waste basket and then the handles can be tied together and the neat ball of waste can be put into the waste container outside the living area.

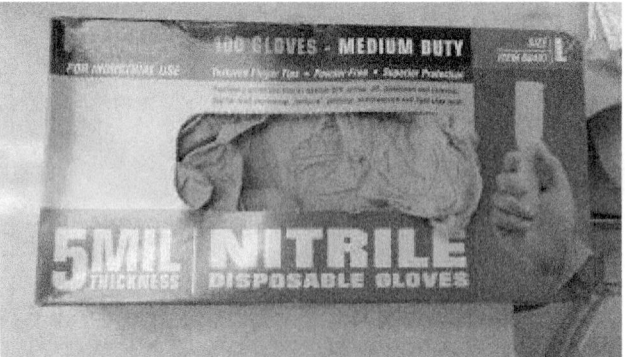

Disposable Gloves

There are a *lot* in a pack and they hold up and don't break. I have even rinsed them off, hung them to dry, and re-used them on occasion.

Cleaning Supplies

I use vinegar and water in a spritzer and a supply of rags.

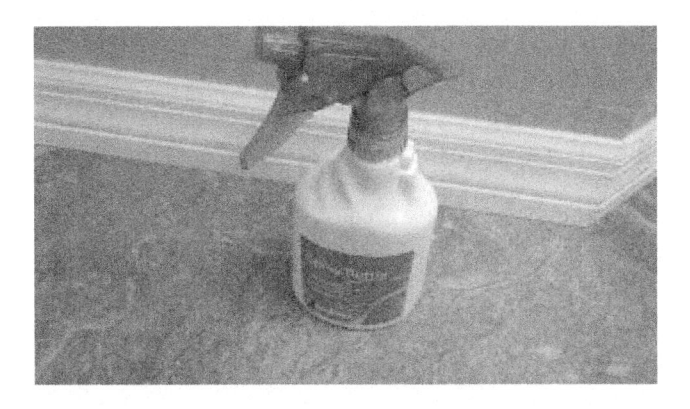

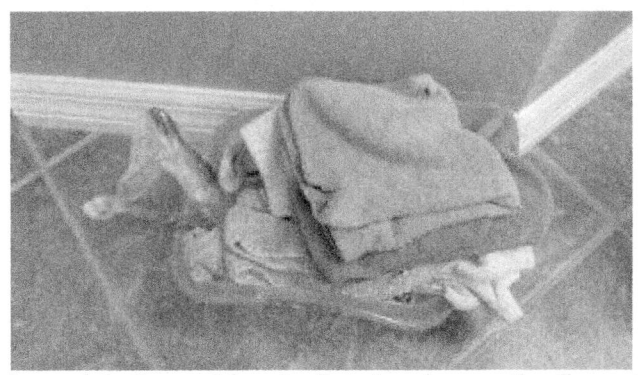

I keep them right by and handy for cleaning up the floor, toilet and sink after a mess.

Deodorizer

I use a clean light Febreze. I hate perfumes even more than the smell of pooh. This scent and brand does the trick and doesn't trigger an asthma attack.

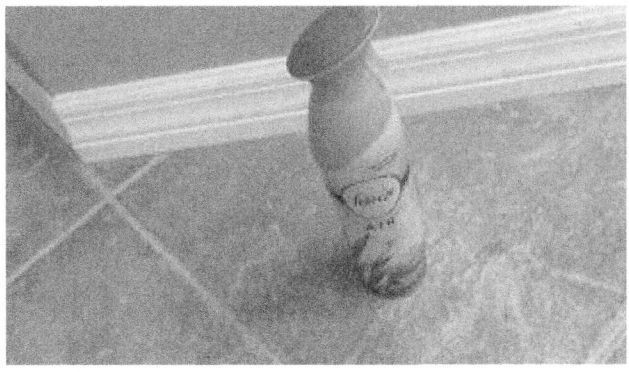

Other Stuff

Bubbles, balls, fidget spinner, tooth pick... anything for George to play with while I am cleaning. Just so he isn't putting his fingers in places and making the mess worse.

To-Go Bags

I keep a bag of wipes, clean shorts, Depends and plastic bags in an oversized purse I can take in the car and into homes and meetings. I also keep a bag of the supplies on his trike.

Step by Step

So this is how we do it.

I have him follow me into the bathroom.
I tell him we are going to check his pants (or change his pants).
I have him lean his backside against his sink which has a counter on one side and a wall on the other so he has stuff to hang onto if he starts to fall. Also, the counter is easier to clean than the wall.

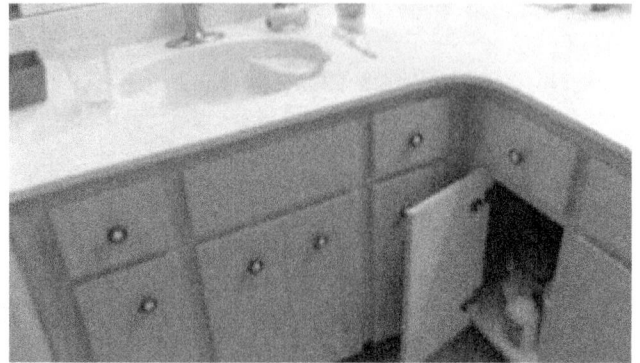

I say, "Take off your shoes." (Sometimes I help him, depending on his balance or ability at the moment.)
I say, "Take off your socks."

I say, "Take off your shorts." Sometimes, if he hesitates, I tease him because I am his wife and can do that. Or I might say, "Drop your pants."

I take his shoes, socks and shorts and toss them into a far corner so they don't get dirty.

I have him turn around now and face the sink. This is also how I have instructed the caregiver to do it so as to protect his modesty or dignity if he has any left.

I gave up trying to have him sit on the toilet and scoot up so I can reach behind him. I have already had to have the toilet re-seated because of the abuse of him flopping down onto the toilet and then trying to move around on it. Besides, reaching back there is hard on my back.

If I see there is poop, I might toss some things into his sink to occupy him while I work.

While he is undressing I put on the gloves and remove anything from the counter (toothbrushes and such) that I want to make sure don't get contaminated.

I place the wipes and the waste basket next to me.

George's sense of time is messed up and he usually wants to put the new pants on after each wipe. I keep reminding him "I am not done yet, stay still."

I take a wipe and put it on top of the pooh and fold the back of the diaper in over the pooh and push the pants down to the floor and he steps out. Sometimes I have him step his legs wider if they are too close together to avoid messing up his legs on the way down. The pants go in the waste basket.

I then scoop with the wet wipes and dump those in the trash.

Usually I get a wet wipe wet and put soap on it and scrub to get all the goo off the skin and hair. Soap is magic! It dissolves the sticky pooh. It took a while to learn this simple fact. Remember, soap dissolves pooh.

As I am working, some crumbs end up on the floor. High fiber diets are pretty flakey. I use the wet wipes to clean that up before he steps in it. (I can clean it better with the cleaning supplies later.)

It helps to have a floor surface that isn't slippery when wet.

I keep the pants out of reach until I am done. Then I hand him a fresh pair of Depends, sometimes I help him get his feet into them and he pulls them up.

After he is dressed I celebrate, "Yay! All clean!" and give him a kiss.

I get him occupied and then I go back in to spritz and wipe surfaces. DONE!

Now as you can tell, George is easy. If your person is mean or more stubborn, you may have to find other methods.

Instructing Respite Caregivers

We have a woman come spend time with George on Tuesdays and Thursdays. Until recently she had not changed his diaper. She would ask him if he wanted help cleaning up or help going to the restroom and George would say, "No."

I told her, "Don't ask for permission. Tell him like I do. After a walk say; 'Let's go right into the bathroom and clean up.'"

I then instructed her in how we do it so she could do it the same way.

Now she checks and cleans.

We are progressing.

More of Living - Good Ol' Days

December 26, 2017

Each day I remind myself, "This is one of the good ol' days."
Life is good right now.

In a caregiver training class we were told to write down in a journal each night three or four emotions we experienced that day.

What I found out is I can have sorrow and joy, silly fun, peace and frustration all in the same day. This may have been the big reason for the exercise. So that we can see for ourselves that it may feel like a struggle one minute and turn around and be funny and fun the next.

It has been so long since I last got a chunk of time long enough to blog. Respite time has been used to exercise, socialize, do paper work, make phone calls, and stuff....

I miss writing to you. It is a way for me to peek at our lives from the outside and to keep you posted on our progress.

Alzheimer's Disease Kills

Our good friend for well over 30 years passed recently from Alzheimer's. He was diagnosed with dementia shortly before George. I am grateful that they showed us the way it can be done.

Karl's strong and wonderful wife, Kathi, was able to care for him all the way through his illness. Karl was not violent through his illness; though he could get cranky, he was also loving. He gave us a big smile of recognition and a hug when we stopped to see him and Kathi on our "Escape Hurricane Irma" trip.

In the last months, Karl was having a type of seizure that I learned is common in Alzheimer's patients. He would be like in a coma. Sometimes a part of his body would be moving, but no one could bring him into conscious interaction. Then, exhausted, he would sleep for hours after the seizure. In the last month or two he was only awake about four hours a day. In the last week or so he was unable to eat and started to fall more often. Once on hospice at home he only lasted a few days and slipped from this world in his sleep.

We all have to leave this world at some point. Knowing thism we still grieve and miss those who go before us.

Memory Care Decisions

Some of those in our support group have spouses who are constantly leaving the house, being agitated, or angry and uncontrollable. These loving caregivers have had to put their spouses into Memory Care units in Assisted Living Facilities in the last two months.

It is heart-wrenching to see these caregivers deal with the agony of having to make such a tough decision. Their hearts break each time they see their loved one who is crying or begging to be taken home. When your loved one does not allow you to sleep at night or is so agitated that they do not cooperate with you in their care, it is a decision that many loving caretakers have to make. The grief is so littered with guilt for not being able to be super human and make their loved one's life better, happier, smoother.

Seeking Income Production

Below is a picture of our Renter, Tirso. He was laid off from his work project and moved out in early November.

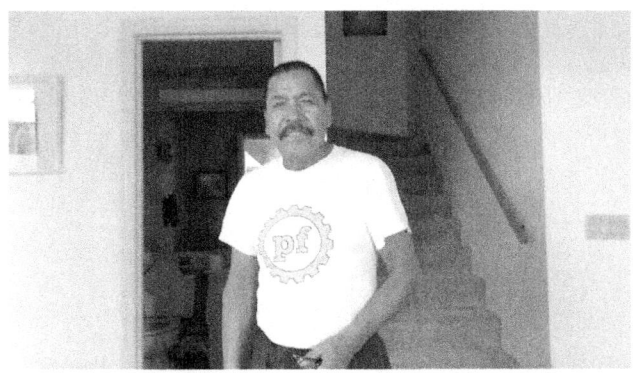

Our other renter moved out after getting so sick that she was unable to work and needed to be with family.

Having empty rooms for a while was fine with me. It was a little less stress and a chance to be on our own. We were expecting visitors this winter so I am keeping one guestroom open and ready for our guests.

Just before Christmas I posted one of our rooms for rent on Craigslist, but so far I have not heard from any good candidates.

Our friend Marsha called me this fall. She said, "I can pay Uber $100 bucks to pick me up at the airport, or I can pay you."

I said, "Where and when should I pick you up?"

Since then I have driven people to and from the airport with and without George at my side. This is a wonderful thing I can do with him; he rides along very calmly and quietly.

Life is good!

George and I still go for walks. He can still walk one to two miles, though sometimes he starts out fast and then sloooows waaaay doooown. When he gets like that, I have to make him stop and rest. He so wants to go. He says, "Ready to go?... Want to walk further?"

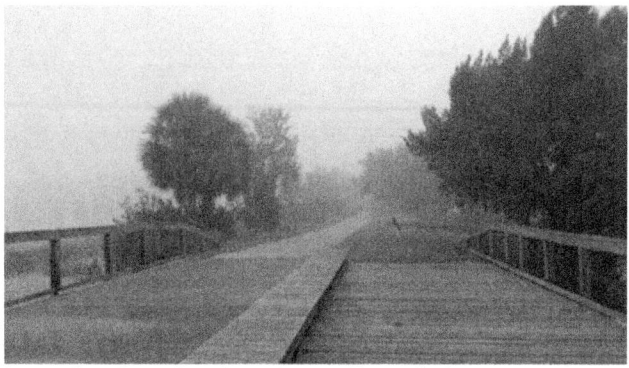

We are in such a lovely place to walk and sit.

We went to the dentist for our annual checkup and I learned that George had broken a tooth and filling. He said it didn't hurt.

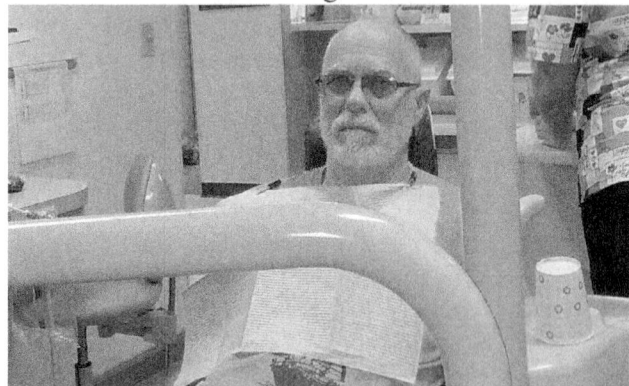

George still likes to go to the old car shows. We met Debra and Glen at the show this fall and George could not sit. He kept on wanting to go back again and look at the cars.

Halloween time was fun. We attended a potluck at our old neighborhood. I get to re-connect with our friends there and enjoy some great cooking.

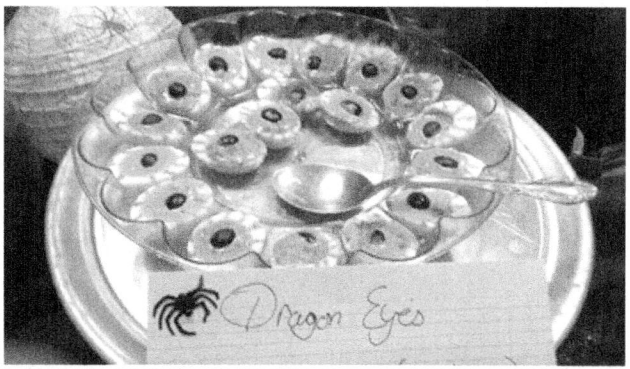

George still bikes, though I have utilized a few respite days to go for rides when I don't have to worry about him at intersections or if he is keeping up or if he needs to change his pants....

Our friends John and Sandy from Wisconsin came to visit. They stayed with us and we had a great time! One night we had our friends Glen and Debra over for dinner while John and Sandy were here.

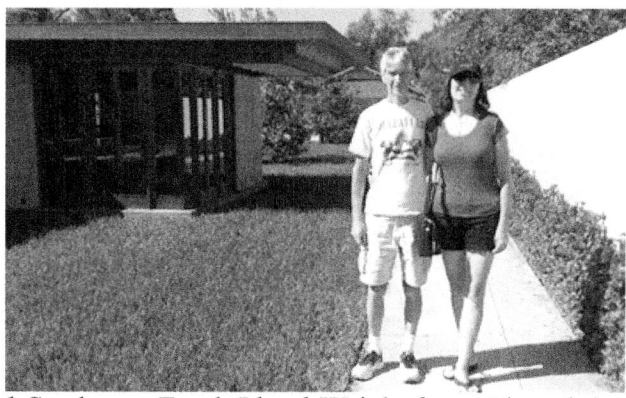

John and Sandy are Frank Lloyd Wright fans. I heard there was a cluster of buildings on a college campus in Lakeland, Florida. On a day that I had a full day of respite, (George was at Key Training Adult Day Care), I drove them over to the campus.

On the way to Lakeland we passed a place selling travel campers. Sandy and John are dreaming of a day they can travel the country. I was dreaming of a time when I was traveling on my own after George passes. So we stopped to take a look.

I got excited about this little trailer. It had room to put my trike and maybe a bike or kayak inside. The bed/couch folds up.

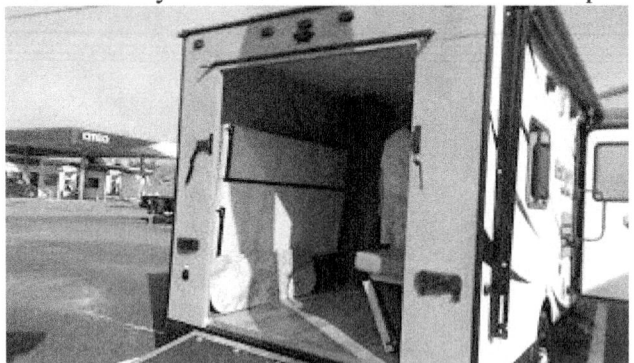

My current van tows about 3,500 lbs. This might work... but a lot more thinking and investigating and dreaming needs to go on.

We took John and Sandy to The Villages for dancing. We invited our bike friends and neighbors Arianne and John to join us. They are ballroom dancers and go dancing three times a week. We had fun watching them.

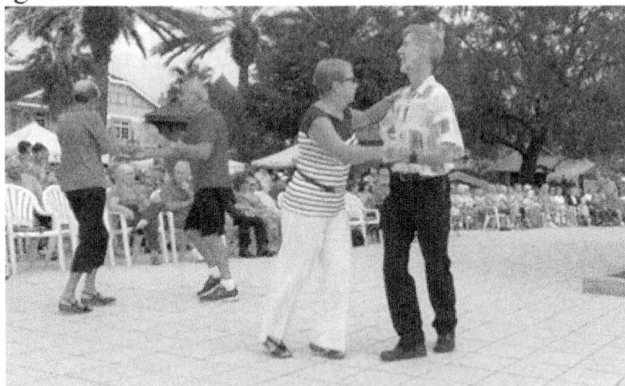

John saw me struggling when I danced with George. I would want to get carried away with the music, but George wants to mirror my movements and can't. I end up going back to rocking side to side like George. John got up and rocked with George so I could get my groove on.

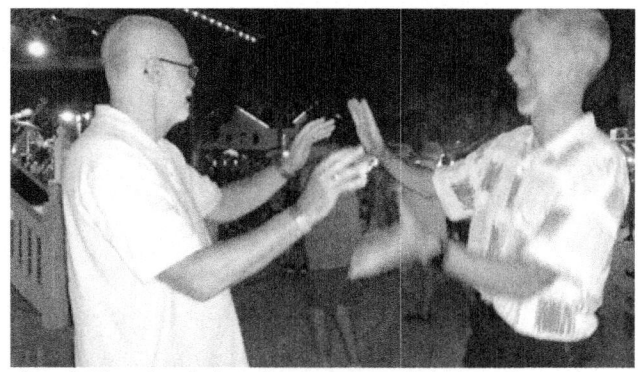

The week of Thanksgiving I went to pick up George at the Key Center and he was proudly wearing a hat he had made... a turkey hat. I laughed.

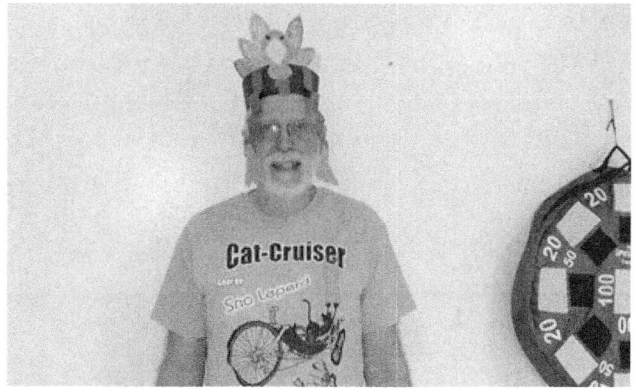

Glen and Debra were celebrating their anniversary and birthdays by spending a few days in Dunedin, FL. It is about a two-hour drive. George and I were joining them for a day of biking and staying one night in a motel. We couldn't leave town until George had his dental cap work done.

We headed to the dentist for 1.5 hours of work to get his tooth ready for a cap. I sat in the room with him to help keep him calm.

After we left the dentist we drove about 1/2 an hour to a picnic area to eat a picnic lunch. We sat down at a picnic table. I pulled out our sandwiches and salad and was enjoying my meal.

I look over and George's lip and tongue are bloody. George keeps chewing on his lip!

I had forgotten about the lip and tongue being numb from the dentist. At first I am gently telling him to not bite his lip. I gently explain the numb lip.

He keeps chewing as if his lip were a piece of tough meat.

Stop it! I explain what is happening again. He doesn't stop.

I put my finger on his lip and try to pull it out from between his teeth. He won't let go.

I am getting hysterical now; yelling at him. "Let go! You are biting your lip!" I yell. "Stop it!" I take the food away.

He keeps chewing his bloody lip. I slap his face thinking it will wake him up from this fog and obsession. He is taking his hand now and pushing the lip so he can bite it better. I gently pull his hand away. He pulls his hand out of my grasp and pushes his lip in so he can bite it. I probably go through 10 different strategies in 20 seconds. I yell, I slap his hands, I cry, I plead, I try to distract. It makes no difference. I feel *really* bad for slapping him. I am not doing this right. I don't know how to break the pattern. Nothing works.

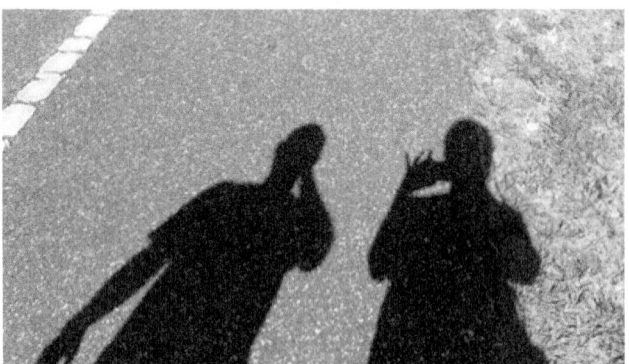

I take him for a walk because my yelling has us both agitated and we both have to calm down, but even as he walks he continues to suck and chew on his lip. He is pushing the lip into his mouth, sucking, making sucky-sounds.

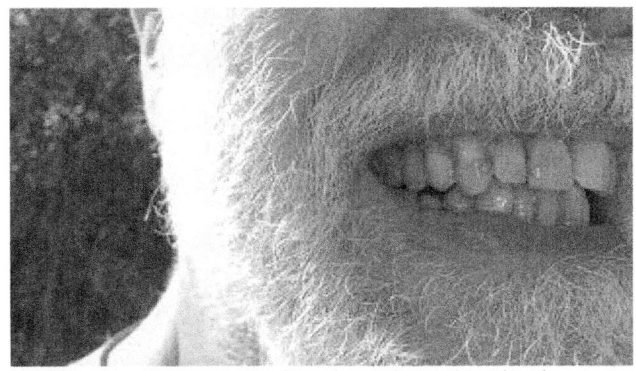

I pack up the remains of our lunch and we get in the car. George continues to suck. The sucky noise is driving me nuts. I lecture, I show him the mirror. He sucks and touches. I ask him if he wants an aspirin or something. He nods yes. When I get a chance I pull off the highway and into a store where I can get a painkiller. I give one to George. A bit later he stops sucking and doesn't mess with his lip again. Sigh.

In Dunedin we meet up with Debra and Glen and spend time helping them celebrate birthdays and their anniversary. The first night we dined at a Mexican Restaurant and laughed a lot.

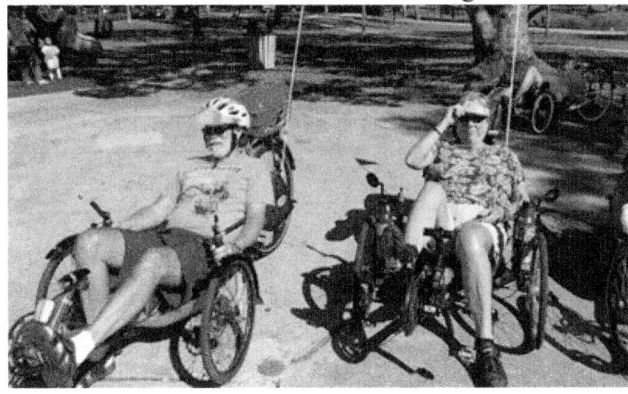

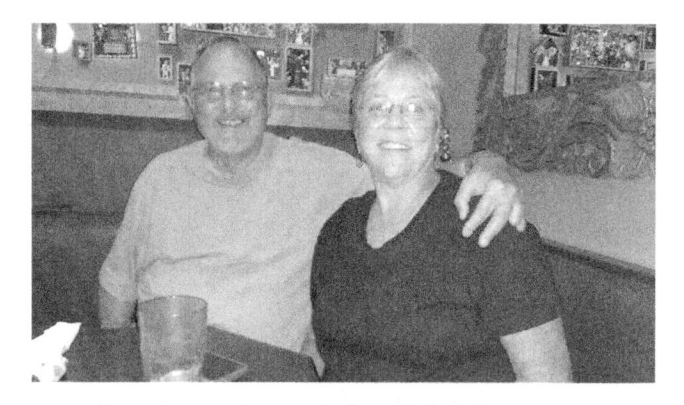

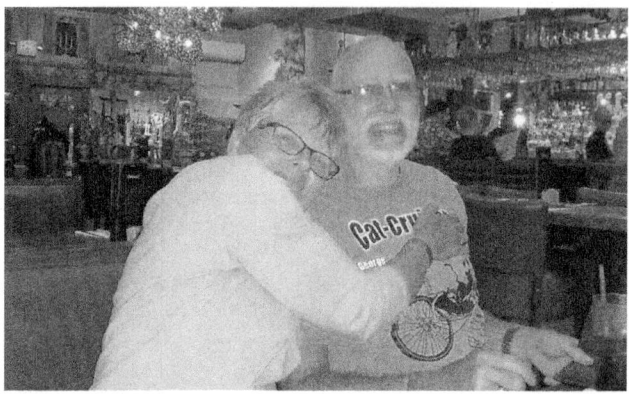

It has been a while since I shared a room with George (our Hurricane escape was the last time). He was up a lot during the night to use the bathroom. Each time I had to get up with him to coach him to wait until he got to the bathroom to pull down his pants. I didn't get much sleep.

The next day we ride the trail. I was worried about George riding the Pinellas Trail because it is an urban trail with a *lot* of road crossings. It turns out that a lot of the road/bike trail intersections are four-way stops. So the cars stop to let us through. Yeah! Glen and Debra helped me keep an eye on George. It turned out to be a beautiful day and a fun ride.

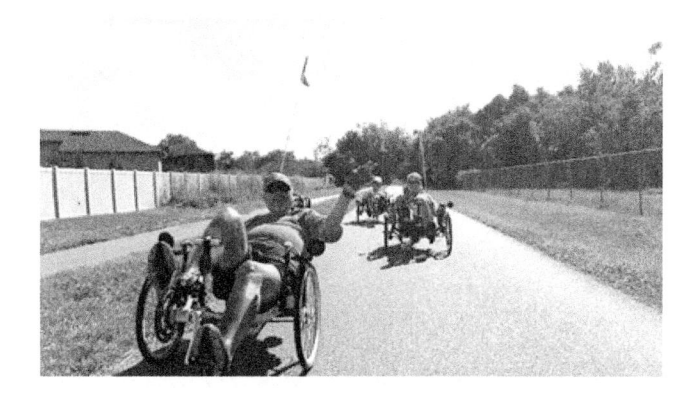

In the News

Some reporter was doing a story on recumbents and came to the Withlacoochee State Trail to get pictures and took our picture. We ended up on the front page of the *Citrus County Chronicle*.

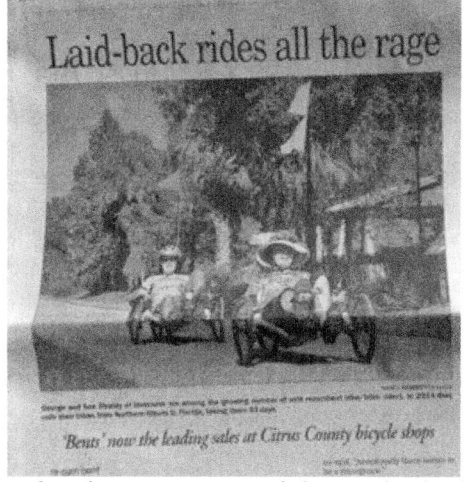

When George's daughter came to visit we invited some friends over for dinner. Northern friends who are only here in the winter are returning to Florida and we are having fun re-connecting.

I bought the game Left Center Right. It is simple and George was able to play it. But my brain is not clear on which dinner party it was that we played it. Sometimes I worry about my brain and memory. My mom died of Alzheimer's disease at 93. This is another reason to blog more often. To record my memories before they get jumbled together.

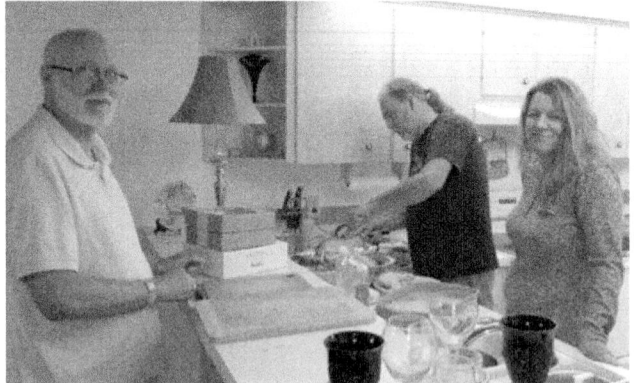

George's daughter wanted to visit the park where George and I got lost and spent the night on the trail a few years ago. I drove them out to Potts Preserve and we walked in only a mile or so. George was walking quite slowly and leaning on the way back out even though we stopped several times to let him rest.

I finally got a call from the VA which arranged for a caregiver who will come for the first time in December and then twice a month, six hours at a time. So I am working on a schedule. I now have respite care three or four days a week! Sometimes for four hours, sometimes six.

Life is good.

AAAAAAhhhhhhhhhh

January 1, 2018

There, a primal scream released in honor of all our caregiver friends. The stress is building like steam in a cooker. Wish I had a convenient little button to push to let it all out.

I sleep in the den. In the morning I get up and pack up my sheet and blanket and put the couch back together. I go into the kitchen and get the coffee started.

Once, I tried to do a few more things before I went to wake George, but then he got up and got dressed and was standing by the bed when I went in... Probably cognitive enough in the early morning to know I needed to turn off the alarm before he could open the door. So this morning I just do the coffee and then I turn off the alarm on his bedroom door and walk in.

He is lying on his side. His torso and legs make a 90-degree angle. This is how he sleeps now; it is a good thing I am not trying to share his bed.

I go into the bathroom and turn on the light. The floor looks like the toilet sprung a leak. There is a pool of urine spreading four feet in front and to the sides of the toilet. I have to do my morning pee. I should have done it in the guest bathroom before coming to wake George. I grab a micro towel and start soaking up the mess.

George gets up and walks by me and stands in the puddle and pees into the toilet.

I rinse the rag and set it outside the puddle and have him step on it before stepping onto the bedroom carpet.

I finish cleaning up the puddle before I finally relieve myself. I tell myself, "Next time pee before you come in to wake George."

I am learning all the time.

VA Provides Supplies!!!

At the support group I learned that incontinence supplies are supplied by the VA. All I have to do is ask George's VA doctor for what I want. So I did and we got two cases of pull-ups on our doorstep. Also a case of gloves and a case of disposable bed pads arrived. YEAH!

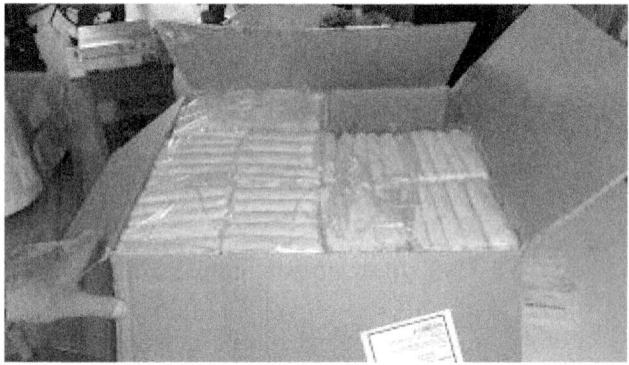

I am finding the pull-ups are *not* as absorbent as the commercial kind. I have purchased some women's extra absorbent menstrual pads to add to his pull-ups when he is at the Key or at night.

The VA-supplied gloves are longer up the wrist and heavy duty. I like them except they are individually wrapped so it is harder to just grab a pair quickly and seems super wasteful. I don't need surgical gloves, I just need disposable gloves to keep the poop out from under my nails and any wounds I might have.

At the Key Center they were telling me he doesn't pee when they take him to the bathroom, but then he overflows his shorts. I instructed them to just have him change his pants at lunch time. "You will have less laundry to do that way," I tell them. I worry that since he rarely goes in the toilet on his own, they may say to me one day that he can no longer go to the Key. That would be a big bummer.

Our friends Nancy and Don are also living with Don's Alzheimer's. Nancy was going to be driving to Brooksville to the store and offered to take George along so I could get a couple hours at home to get stuff done. What amazing friends we have!

And my sister!! She sent us a big box. When I went to open it there was a paper over the contents saying "Don't open until December 14th."

I waited and when December 14th came I pulled off the cover and there were 12 gifts inside all wrapped in Christmas Paper and numbered for the 12 days of Christmas. What a thoughtful thing to do! I enjoyed opening one gift a day.

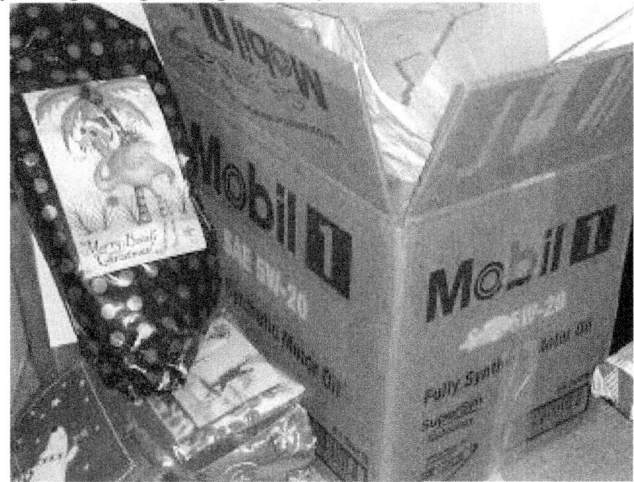

Christmas Eve I held my traditional potluck party with friends. I was more worried about this one than ever before. It is usually no sweat, but I worried that George would follow me all over the house and try to help while I was getting the place ready. To the rescue, Debra and Glen offered to watch him while I got ready for the party. Yeah! And then friends pitched in to keep him settled during dinner so he wasn't up getting 20 servings and using the serving utensils to eat and sneezing on the food.

We had a great time. Even Connie (the woman who broke both ankles) came… in a wheelchair, with one foot propped up.

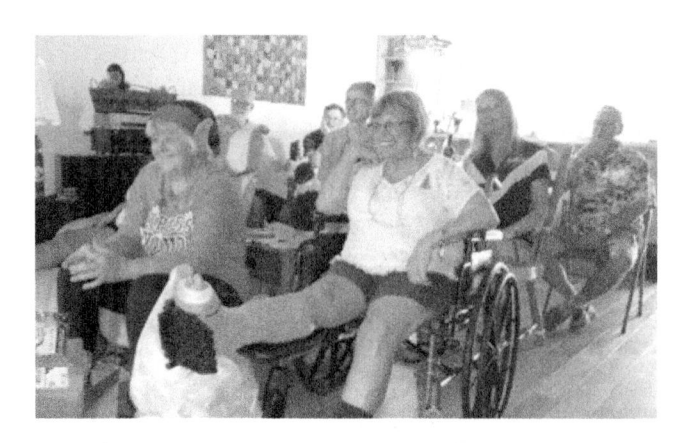

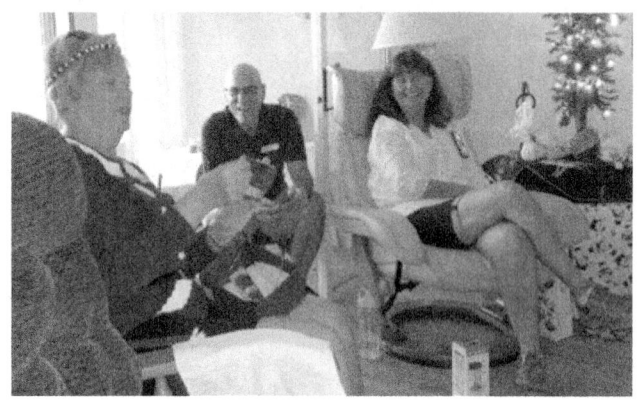

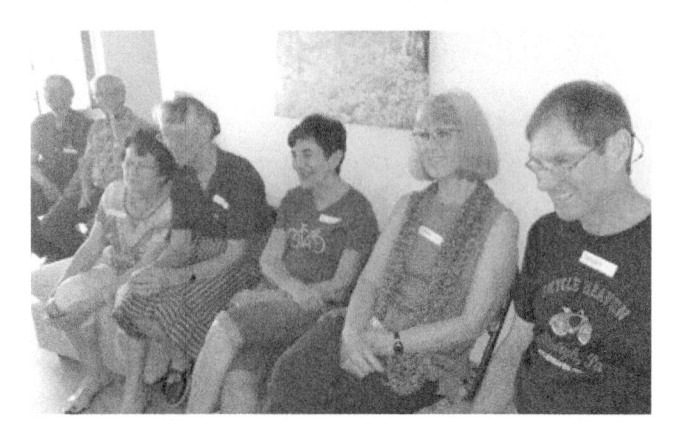

SUSAN STRALEY

Christmas Day we went to our old neighborhood and dined with Louise and Richard, Debra and Glen. George kept going back up for food. Even when his plate was half full he was getting up to get more food.

After dinner he was going up to get his second helping of dessert and began sneezing all over the food on the buffet. Argh!

New Year's Eve we went to our old neighborhood clubhouse to celebrate. It was great chatting with our friends and neighbors from there. However, I had trouble keeping George away from the buffet table again. When I sat down to play Rummikub he tried to eat the cubes. He kept me hopping up to chase him down or get more stuff for him most of the evening.

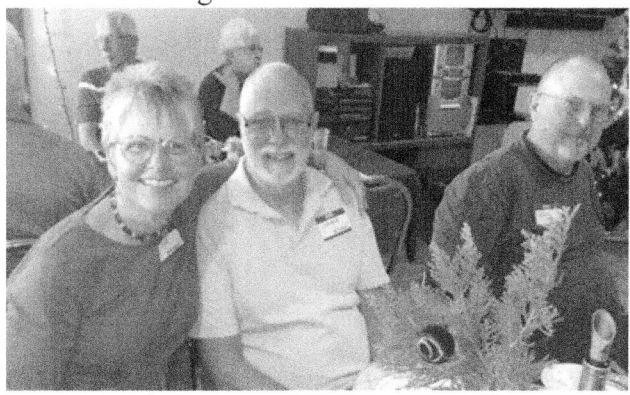

Changes

I am now trying to learn about tandem trikes and the choices out there. It is getting too dangerous for George to trike. He has stopped in the middle of intersections, and has a hard time getting going from a stop because he is in the wrong gear all the time.

One day we are sitting at the dinner table eating. George keeps looking at me and looking out the window. Then when I look at him he says, "I am looking for my wife to come." I paused to absorb that, then I said, "Oh, that's nice!" and he looked right at me and smiled.

Sleep, the Game Changer

I have an alarm on the bedroom door where George sleeps. I have wondered if it was loud enough to wake me while I am sleeping at the other end of the house. This morning I found out.

The alarm sounded. I got up and I left the den where I had been sleeping wonderfully. I glanced at the digital clock above the kitchen stove. It is 4 a.m.

George is standing outside the bedroom in his pull-ups.

"George, it is the middle of the night," I say, knowing as I say it that I am wasting my breath.

George echoes, "Middle of the night."

I walk past him into the bedroom knowing that he will follow me. The room smells of urine and I know his bed is wet.

He stands in front of the toilet trying to go pee. He is all peed out. He usually is by the time he gets to the toilet. I get a rag soapy and wash and rinse him down as he stands there.

"It's 4 in the morning, George," I tell him. "You have to go back to bed."

But I can tell by his wide-eyed look that isn't going to happen.

As I am taking the wet things off the bed he is putting on his pants and shoes and socks. He goes into the kitchen and fixes his bowl of cereal and eats while I dump the wet things into the washing machine and re-make the bed.

I feel the resentment and frustration. I stuff it. I resign myself to being up for the rest of the day. I have never been one to nap during the day; I can't fall asleep during the day unless I am sick.

It is dark out when George is ready to go for his walk. I have him watch a movie while I drink coffee and read the paper.

At 6 a.m. I grab a flashlight and we go for a walk. I see the neighborhood dog owners walking their dogs and scooping up pooh. I think that what I am doing is similar. I am taking George for a walk to get the contents of his intestines moving.

A fellow Diva had started a Facebook Messenger group for us just yesterday. I go to my phone and report my early rising and resentment. In minutes I get supportive comments.

I remember that this morning we have yoga with friends and then we get to meet with our dementia family over coffee.

I feel fortunate to have so much support around us.

Love Beneath Us

February 2, 2018

Feeling The Love...
I just can't believe how fortunate and blessed we are to be surrounded by wonderful and loving friends.

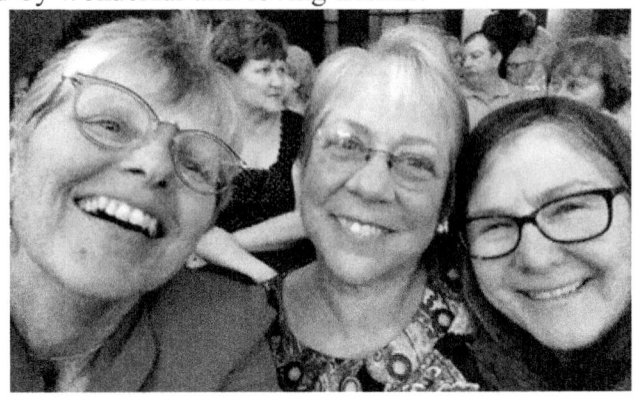

I Get Away!

Early in January I was able to get away from caregiving for three nights, thanks to the Key Center Adult Day Care, friends, and a retired nurse.

The Alzheimer's Organization provided the opportunity with a lobby day in Tallahassee. I set it up so George would be at Day Care for three full days. I reserved a place through Airbnb. It was a two-bedroom apartment in the College district within 1.5 miles of the capital.

I asked three different couples to pick up George from Day Care and bring him home and spend two hours with him.

The Nurse was to show up at 7 and stay until he got on the bus to the Key the next morning.

Glorious freedom! It was a very cold few days but I was able to bike and walk and turn around without having to bump into or care for George. I didn't even call to check on him.

On the way up to Tallahassee I walked at Manatee Springs and biked a bit of the St. Marks Trail.

The next day I biked around Tallahassee and sat and read a book.

In the evening I rode my bike to the capital for an Alzheimer's Awareness Rally.

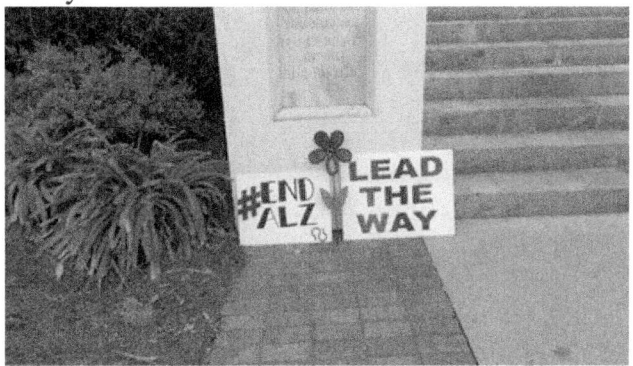

There I met up with my friend and fellow Dementia Diva, Dianne.

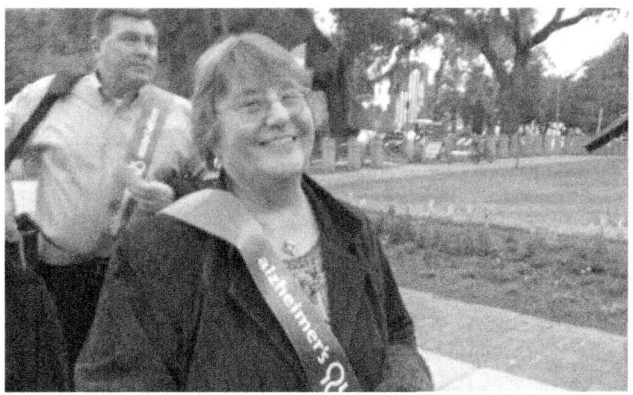

I loved my apartment. It cost me less than the area motels and was close to shops and restaurants and trails.

Thanks to Jennifer and Dave, Mari and Jerry, Frankie and Dennis, Debra and Glen for picking up George from The Key Center Adult Day Care, feeding and entertaining him so I could get away.

231

Tandem Love

The last time I wrote I mentioned I was searching for a tandem.

I got a call from our friends, Bill and Christine around Christmas time offering to purchase for George an electric assist for his trike. WOW! I was so moved I began to cry. Bill said he would like to see George continue to bike as long as possible.

I thought about it long and hard because, though George is slowing down on his trike, adding speed might be more dangerous for him, other bikers, and motorists. Yet it would be great to go faster and keep riding with our community of biking friends.

Lately I have missed riding with the group because George can't keep up or I have to stop to help George across the streets.

I searched for a tandem.

Our friend Cindy offered to let us use her Greenspeed Anura for as long as George could ride. Cool! Thank you, Cindy!

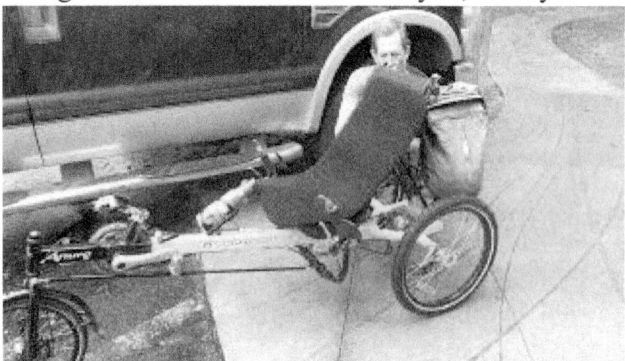

This is a trike with two wheels in the back. It can hook onto another Greenspeed Anura to make a tandem. She and her husband Regis helped us experience the tandem by hooking up two trikes for us. Thank you, Regis! It seemed slow and heavy. I didn't think we would be able to keep up with the group. Argh! The price of a trike *and* electric assist was way too much!

We have lived our lives trying hard to be not only self-sufficient but to be in a place to help others. So accepting gifts from others now takes changes in thought. It took agonizing weeks of trying to find an option that would work for the least amount of money. I mean, really, how much longer will George be able to bike?

Should I spend the money?

Will I regret *not* doing something so he (we) can bike longer?

Am I making an emotional and foolish purchase?

I don't want to let go of my biking partner, but the reality is he is leaving this world and I am staying behind. He doesn't understand time and I don't know that he is aware that he is missing biking opportunities.

But then I thought of being able to zoom here and there again on my bike even while I am caregiving, and the thought thrills me. Run to the store, no problem. Go 40 miles, no problem.

To be able to keep up with our community of bikers and still socialize and ride two or three times a week would give me great joy.

I enlisted the help of our friend Glen to help me search for another delta trike. Thank you, Glen!

Glen found a Greenspeed Anura, at the Hostel Shoppe in Wisconsin. I went to order it and then thought that maybe I should just let our friend Rolf know what I am up to. Rolf owns the Hostel Shoppe; maybe he could provide a coupon or discount. Rolf and George had biked together and enjoyed each other's company. Rolf went beyond a coupon. Thank you, Rolf!

Today I got an email from Bill D. He said he has ordered the electric assist! I am so excited!

What a love story! This is the Withlacoochee Bicycle Rider community working to keep George and me on the trail riding as long as possible. Thank you to everyone who is helping make this possible. I had never dreamed 10 years ago when we started riding with you that we were becoming part of such a generous and supportive community of friends. I feel the love!

SUSAN STRALEY

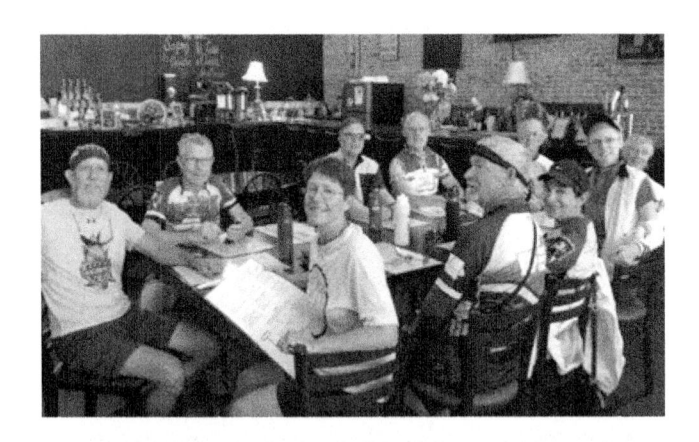

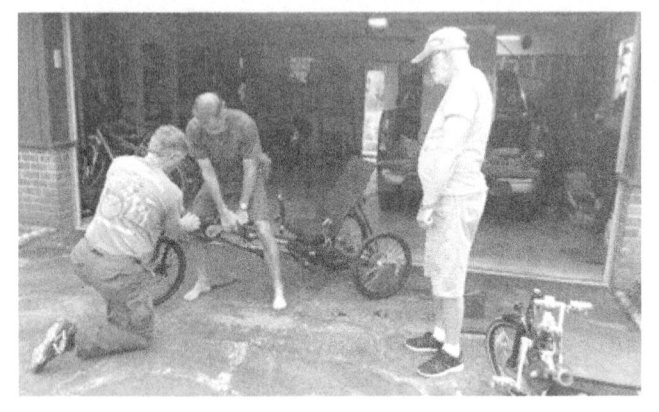

Our First E-assist Tandem Rides

February 13, 2018

We rode our trikes down to Floral City on Sunday, February 11. We were riding down on our old trikes and would ride back on our new electric assist tandem.

It was a rough morning with George. It was also sad to know that this would be George's last ride on his beloved orange, custom-painted Catrike.

As we rode, I cried, sucking it up and wiping away the tears whenever I saw someone about to pass.

Then our friend Jennifer pulled up beside me. She was there, she said, to ride with us on this special occasion and to escort us on our first tandem ride home. What a wonderful sweet gesture!

We pulled off the trail on the street where Regis and Cindy live. Lined up on their driveway were several of our bike friends. They were waiting to see us try our new trikes for the first time.

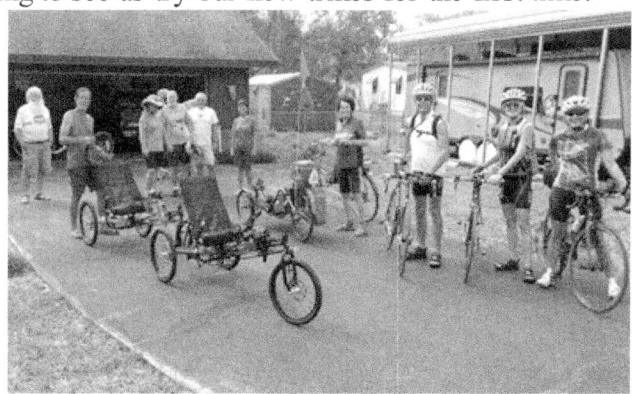

Our friends have been unbelievably awesome! Regis had a lot of puzzles to solve on the trike. He added a bracket to hold the battery for the electric assist. He added bottle holders and designed a holder for the assist controls. It looked wonderful.

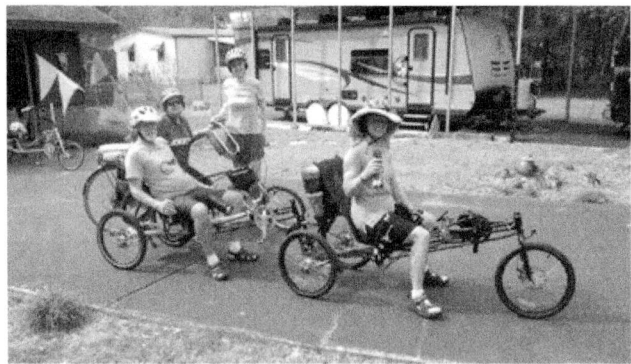

After I took a test ride, we put George on the back and headed home. Regis and Cindy, Louise and Richard, and Jennifer rode with us. Also Larry Varney an editor at Bentrideronline was visiting Cindy and Regis and rode with us too. (Bentrideronline.com is an online magazine dedicated to recumbent bikes.)

Every time I looked in the rearview mirror I saw that George was smiling.

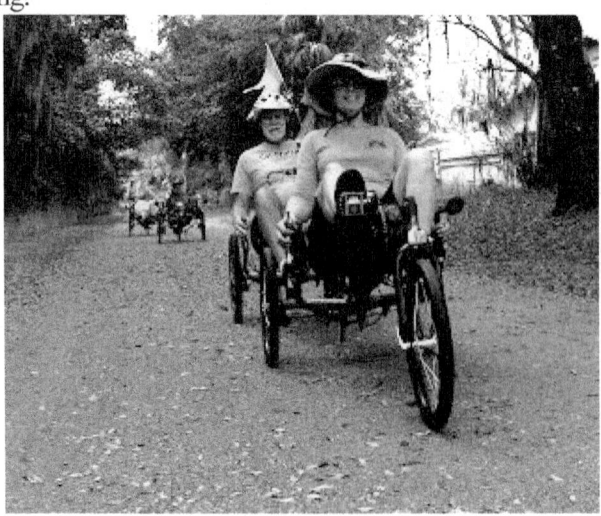

Group Ride Number One

Our first group ride was Tuesday, February 13, 2018. The weather report was for rain. I was worried. I was so looking forward to riding with the group and seeing how we did in the group with the tandem trike. Can we keep the same pace?

Ride time arrived and though the skies were grey I backed the long bike out of the garage and we headed out, getting used to the different levels of assist and how it works with the gearing.

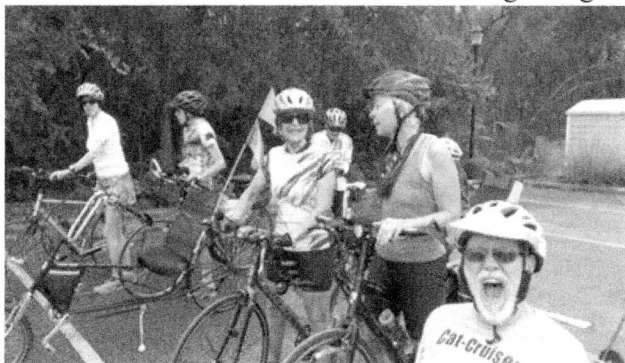

We met the group as we usually do at Wallace Brooks Park. Ride time came and we were on our way north on the Withlacoochee Trail. I tried to find a good speed. It seemed that level one power wasn't enough. I struggled to keep up with the group. Level two was too much: I kept having to coast to stay back with the group.

We hadn't gone a mile when I started sensing something was wrong. The front wheel or my handlebar or both would turn for no reason.

The handles I hang on to and use for steering run underneath my seat and are perpendicular to the boom when the front wheel is straight forward. There is a rod that runs from my steering bar (handlebar) to the front wheel.

I would be riding along and all of a sudden my handlebar would turn 45 degrees. Sometimes the front wheel would suddenly turn.

We stopped once or twice on the way up and someone helped tighten the rod that ran from the front wheel to the handlebar, thinking that would fix it. But it didn't!

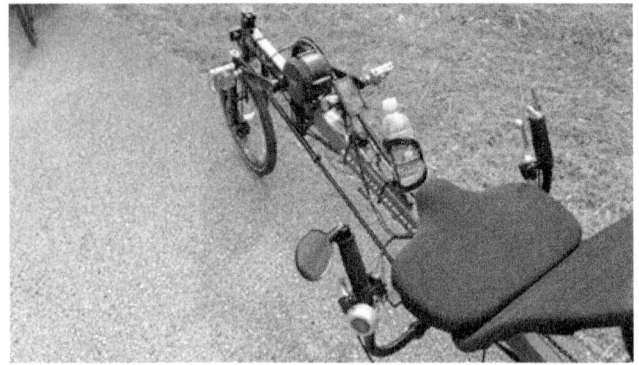

We arrived at our halfway rest stop in Citrus Springs. Here we gather to take a break and chat. Some of the riders gathered around and again tightened the rod, loosened the front wheel pivot post and pumped the front tire which was low.

That should fix it.

We rode on to the Boulevard Bistro restaurant. It was super busy and there was rain in the forecast for the afternoon. I didn't know how the e-assist would tolerate rain. George and I left right away instead of eating there. Everyone else stayed.

On the way south it got harder and harder to pedal. When I shifted in my seat, the steering went catawampus. We were going slower and slower and it was *sooo* hard!

Then the display showed we either weren't creating power or we were out of power....

A fellow Withlacoochee Bicycle Rider came by when I stopped to rest and saw that the front tire was flat. I had not had a chance to buy tubes yet. But we had the whole front wheel from George's trike with us. We put that on.

I discovered that if I held the front wheel straight and pushed down on the steering rod I could put the handlebar back in its correct position. It just didn't make sense!

We were totally out of electric power now. Preston said we were only three miles from Chicken King Restaurant. I needed to rest and hydrate and eat. George looked fresh, but I was whipped.

Finally, around 3:00 we arrived home. The transition from the street to our drive has quite a bump. On our Catrikes, as we approach our driveway we slow down and then make our way carefully over the curb and up the drive. But this time when we hit the curb the front tire turned and we skidded into a bush.

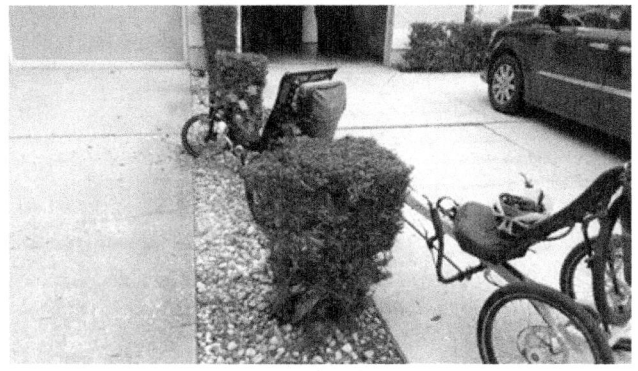

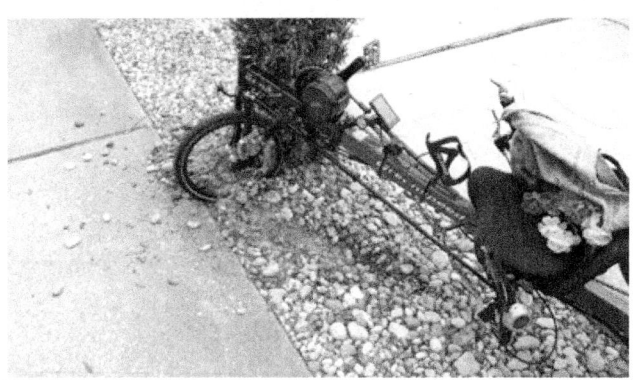

I was glad to be home. I cleaned George and set him in front of a movie before I went back out to straighten the bikes and put them in the garage.

Something needs to be fixed before we head out again.

Back In The Saddle

March 21, 2018

 It was really a downer to have our new tandem trike not function well. I had been dreaming of biking long and far again with the group and on our own. When our first rides went so poorly, I was really discouraged.
 I was able to get the Greenspeed Anuras into our minivan and take them to Trailside.bike in Floral City. Greg is the bike mechanic there with a good reputation for his knowledge and skill repairing recumbent bikes. I was hoping he could fix our new ride.
 The shop was very busy. I filled out a repair form and left the trikes there. Our old trikes were there to get maintenance as well. For the first time in years we were trike-less. ARGHHH!!!!
 After several days our tandem trike was done and I took George out on a ride around the back streets of Inverness. The trike was riding so much better!

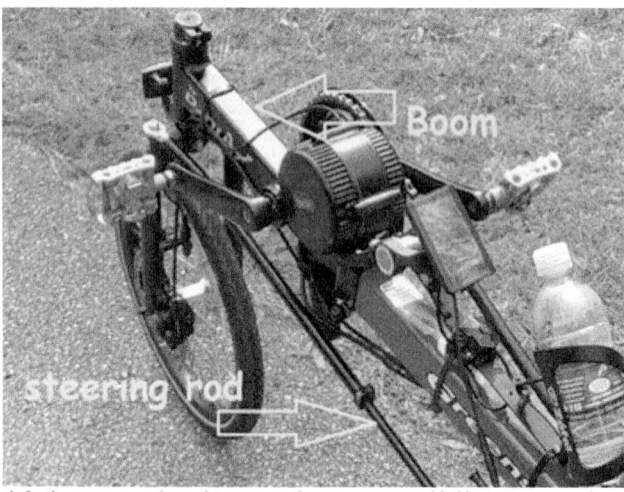

 Greg said it was the boom that was sliding, not the steering mechanism. With all the abuse, the boom had bent. Greg had to take the trike to an automobile machine shop to get the boom straightened. Then to keep the boom from sliding, he added shims. Now the trike is solid and no longer slipping.

On our backstreet ride we went over some rough roads. First my water bottle holder fell off. Then George's would no longer hold his thermos. Then we lost a reflector.

I was so frustrated. We went home. I set George up to watch a movie and I went outside to put the tandem in the garage.

I called our friend Richard about the stuff falling off and right away he dropped everything and came over. He fixed it! Thank you, Richard.

On Saturday, March 17, I took George for a ride and nothing fell off and the trikes were solid and rode so well that we kept going and going. We ended up riding almost 50 miles that day. Then the next day we rode with friends up to Swampy's in Dunnellon. We rode over 91 miles in two days! Often I would look back and George would be smiling and many times he would be pedaling. How's that for a 70-year-old man with late-middle stages of Alzheimer's!

I am amazed that even as unsteady on his feet he can be, he can lift his foot over the boom to get on his trike without hanging on to anything. Yet at home when we walk in and I ask him to stomp his feet on the rug and demonstrate it to him, he can't lift his foot an inch off the floor.

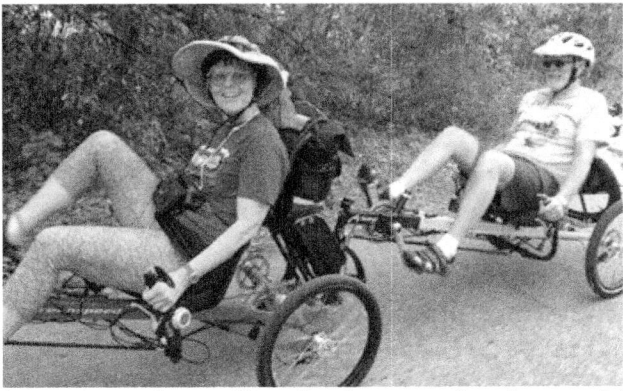

I love the new tandem trike. It gives us freedom to bike with friends again. I think this part of George... this trike riding with the group part of George... is still there. He is enjoying it. I am enjoying it. Thanks again to all those who contributed to this amazing project!

Support Group

On Mondays we go to a support group called "Memory Lane." It is sponsored and organized by the First United Methodist Church in Homosassa, FL. This is where I met the gals who became the Dementia Divas with me. We are women caring for spouses and others with dementia. Though since we started calling ourselves the Divas, some men caregivers have joined in. So now we are the Dementia Divas and Amazing Princes.

We meet every week, unlike so many support groups that only meet once a month. I think it is because of the regular weekly contact that the group members have gotten close. We are a family of friends now.

The meetings are all the way in Homosassa which is about 35 minutes away. The drive is so worth it. There is good information coming from those more experienced and I get to help others who are starting out in their dementia journey.

There are a group of church volunteers who keep our loved ones occupied in one room so we caregivers can meet and cry and complain and strategize without our loved ones in the room. That is *such* a great idea and *sooo* helpful to us caregivers.

The other day during Memory Lane, I was complaining that I didn't get my coffee until late in the morning. One of the other caregivers suggested I have coffee and relax *before* I go get George up out of bed. WOW! What a difference that makes to a cheerful start to the day. I even started doing the Five Tibetan Rites (exercises) before getting coffee.

And then I learned to put the paper disposable bed pads over the washable ones. Yes, the trash can fills up, but I am not doing laundry every morning. I hope that all caregivers can find a support group to provide them good suggestions, good help, and good hugs.

Dealing With Death

Three of my fellow Dementia Divas have already experienced the death of their loved one. It is surprising to me to have their loved ones passing within the year that I have been with them.

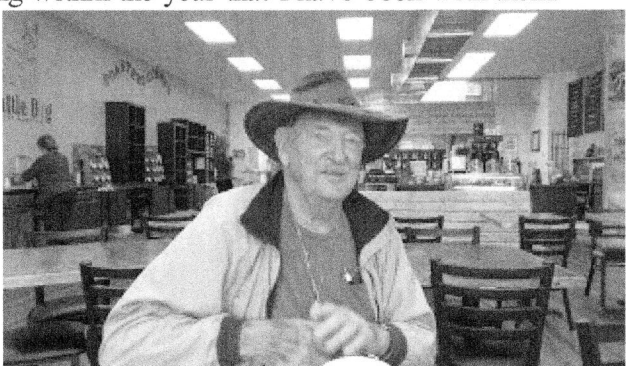

Last night we lost our friend Herb who not only had dementia but had cancer and heart disease. His wife is an amazing, strong, positive, and loving Diva. Herb loved life and had ambitions and just a few months before his passing he, with the help of his wife, published a book about his faith. I offer my condolences to his wife, Dianne, and a hearty "goodbye" to *"the chicken whisperer."*

Symptoms Increase

George is having more times when he is unsteady on his feet. He can't walk as far as he did just a few months ago. If I push it further it takes a long time to get back with lots of rest.

The other day he fell while getting out of a chair and bent the TV tray leg. I ask him if he hurts. He has not reported any injuries.

We were walking a couple blocks to our friend's house to dine and George was really leaning forward on his toes. I kept stopping him and telling him to put weight on his heels. He was drooling as he walked. It must have been very hard for him.

I think I mentioned a day when he didn't recognize me. That isn't all the time. Most of the time he seems to know me and look at me with love still. I am so blessed to have that. My heart would break into a thousand pieces if he was un-trusting and afraid of me.

Progress is not a straight line. For days I was getting up to puddles in his bathroom each morning and a bed soaked with urine. Even with two diapers on and added pads. But lately I have just been using one diaper and he gets up during the night and changes it. His bed isn't as soaked. I have been laying towels on the bathroom floor at bedtime and most of the time in the morning they are dry.

Each morning he gets his own cereal ready and eats it while I am getting dressed. One night I had left grated cheese on the counter. In the morning he had grated cheese covered in milk for his breakfast.

George's Memorial Trike

When Regis was assembling the trike and putting brackets on and stuff, he started an ongoing account at the bike shop. Currently it is called "George's Trike Account." Since then we have had expenses for repairs that were also put on the account. A friend asked how she could help; did we need anything else for the tandem?. When I told her about the account she went down and put money toward the bill. Thank you!

Cindy, who donated one of the trikes on the tandem, suggested that we keep the tandem available to those in our bike group in the years ahead. What a great idea! This tandem will continue to keep on giving long after George is gone. It is a great way for those in our bike group to stay mobile when faced with injury or disease that hinders their ability to bike.

Naming the Trike

Right now we are calling the tandem, "George's trike." But it needs a better, longer-term name.

So far we have had two suggestions:

The Withlacoochee Choo Choo
The Gravy Train

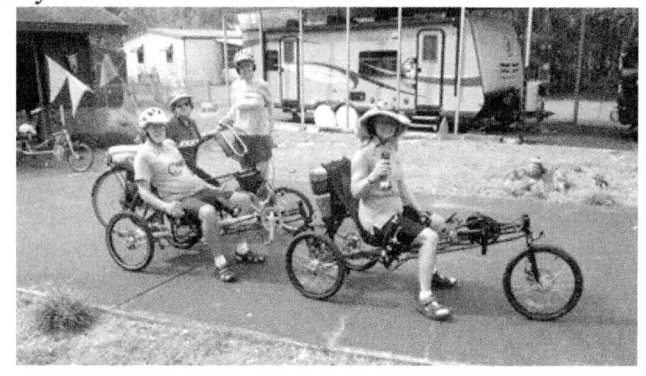

Applause and Tears

April 21, 2018

    I have great news! The other day our friend Bill emailed and told us the bill at the bike shop for the accessories and repairs on the tandem had been paid in full! We are surrounded by angels!
    I am in awe at the support our bike friends have poured on us and how they have gotten behind us. This tandem project is just one of the many ways that individuals have shown their support and kindness.
    When I stopped in the shop to get the bill for the repairs on our old trikes... that too was paid in full!
    WOW!

    On 4/14/2018 we rode the tandem 52 miles. When we got to Ridge Manor we took a break and I took some pictures to commemorate the event.

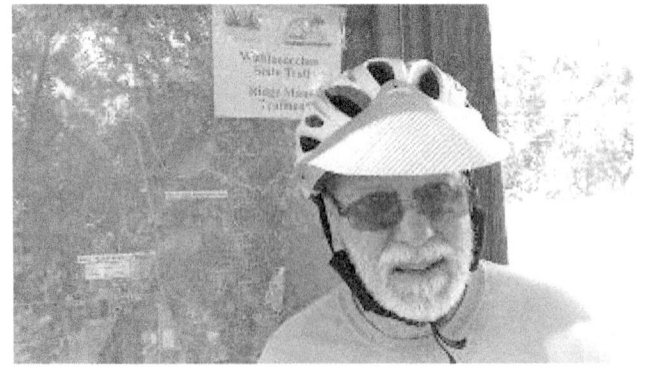

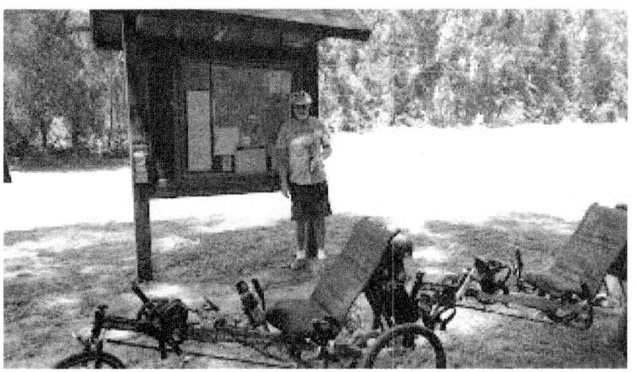

We biked back to Inverness and the "Taste of Inverness" was going on right next to the trail. I had forgotten to pack our tickets. We went home to get them and then I drove us over to the event, parking about 2 blocks away.

It was hot and suddenly George could not walk or stand. One of his legs wouldn't straighten. I sat him down at a table and went in search of food and drink for us. I rushed - I was afraid he might start trying to walk around.

Our friends were there; they were drinking and enjoying the day. I didn't feel I should do that. After feeding and watering George, I held him up as we slowly made it back to a bench by the road. I sat him down and rushed to get the car. I don't know why I rushed, he couldn't go anywhere. I guess I was just concerned he might try to get up and fall down.

Sister Visit

I was sooooo looking forward to my sister's visit. She had visited last year and we had such a great time. We had kayaked and walked and talked. This time she was traveling with her husband, Dave, whom we love. Early in Dave and George's career they had worked for the same small company.

Dave had back surgery a few years ago and has some health issues, so I knew our visit with them would not be active. It would be fun but different, a little less physical movement, maybe some more time sitting around visiting.

I had told them I had two guestrooms upstairs and a bathroom all to themselves. They would be comfortable.

But....

I am always obsessing about my financial future. A few weeks before, I had listed the rooms for rent. I had gotten an inquiry and I had told the person the room would not be available until May (because I wanted to save the rooms for my sister and brother-in-law and for a "gals night" I had planned with a couple of the newly-widowed Dementia Divas). The potential renter said they needed the room sooner than May. So we went our separate ways.

I was second-guessing my decision to keep the rooms open for these two events. Was I making the right decision? I talked to a friend who said to me, "You have to decide your priorities. Is it to have fun or is it to secure your financial future." *Argh!!!* Always the wire I walk!

Then I got an email from Tirso's daughter. (Tirso rented from me last summer and fall.) She said her dad was on his way to Florida for another temporary job and asked if he could rent a room from me again.

Here was another opportunity for me to say yes to a renter. This renter I had already tried and I knew he paid and was neat and quiet. I said in a reply email that, yes, Tirso can return, but the rooms won't be available until May 1st.

Sunday, April 8th, Tirso is standing in my driveway when we return home from somewhere. He drove two days to get here in time. He starts working on Monday, he tells me. He wants to know, can he move in?

I am flustered. I have to get George into the house, cleaned up and occupied; Tirso is waiting for an answer anxiously. I try to explain my dilemma, but there is a language barrier. I try to explain my sister's visit, the ladies night. I am not fluent in Spanish. Tirso is better in English than I am in Spanish but not a whole lot. My brain bounces, stutters... if I turn him away now.... will it hurt Mary and Dave's visit? What will I tell the Divas who are probably looking forward to this break away from their new lives?

I say yes to Tirso and inside I groan. My chest tightens. I may appear like a decisive person to some, but decisions like this are hard.

Tirso moves in some of his things. I text my sister and let her know.

Late afternoon on Monday, April 9th, my sister and Dave arrive. I asked to help haul their things in. She tells me they got a motel room. They weren't comfortable sharing a bathroom with a stranger. I start to cry, then sob. Mary hugs me while I cry. She assures me that they will still come and hang out often. I feel awful. I know I have put a financial burden on them. I am sure they were expecting a comfortable place to stay in my home without the expense of four nights in a motel room. I wanted to show my sister love and I had made the trip more difficult and expensive for her. I regret my decision on the renter. Still, I am surprised by my emotional tears.

We had a nice visit with my sister and Dave.

While George was at Day Care one day, Mary and I got out for a bike ride.

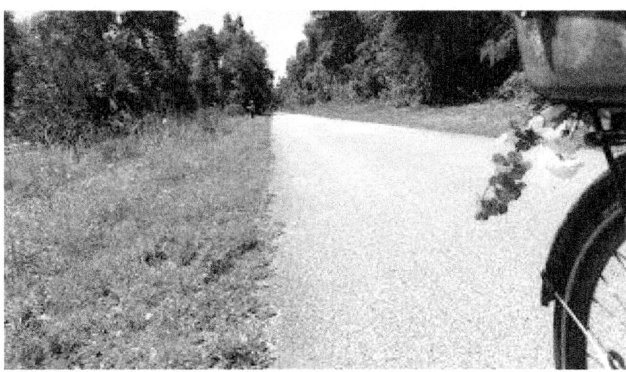

Yes! I got a ride without George trailing behind.

Dave is a handyman and tends to notice things. He noticed I had some lights out in my kitchen. I was not even aware of it. He replaced them for me. Thank you, Dave!

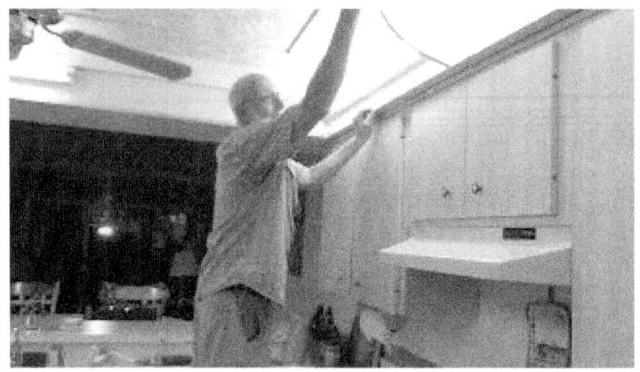

The ladder still stands in the dining room reminding me to put it away. Day after day after day it nags me.

Disease is Nibbling Away

George doesn't talk at all except to mirror what I say. He doesn't understand much. I give him very short commands. But then once in a while in a group, he surprises me by laughing out loud in his old laugh at someone's wisecrack.

I made a video recently of him exercising and put it up on my YouTube channel. (April 2018). Then I looked at the exercise video I took of him in August of 2017. Wow. What a difference eight months can make.

A Not So Typical Morning

March 8, 2018

It is about 7:30 a.m. and dawn is here. I have looked at the headlines, drunk my coffee, made my bed and done a few exercises. Now it is time to "go to work."

I go to George's bedroom (it used to be "ours"). Before I open the door I reach up and turn off the alarm.

I enter and see that George is lying on his back in the bed. Two wet diapers are sitting on the carpeted floor next to the bed.

"Good morning, George," I say and he replies the same.

I check the bathroom and the towels I laid on the floor the night before are dry. *Good*, I think, feeling relief that I don't have to quick-mop the floor before he walks in.

I hear George shake as he stretches. I help George out of bed. He is wobbly and keeps rocking back onto the bed after each attempt to stand.

I make him stand a moment before I guide him to the bathroom. As I guide him I have to keep reminding him to keep his pants up until he gets to the bathroom. He has his thumbs stuck in the front of his pull-ups tugging them downward as he walks stiff-legged to the toilet.

After he pees in the toilet he reaches for his shorts that I have left on the counter the night before. I have left the bathroom to pick up the wet diapers and I have to rush back in to stop him from putting the clean shorts on over his wet diapers. "No, we have to change your wet underwear first," I say.

He keeps trying, I keep saying it differently. "No, pants wet... not yet."

I gesture and tug at his pull-ups. I pull them down for him and he steps out of them. Then he reaches for the shorts. He smells like pee, of course.

I put a towel down, turn on the water in the shower, quickly strip myself, and I guide George into the shower, working around him so

I can grab the shower wand, test the heat of the water, and be between him and the controls and the soap.

I wash him and rinse him while he mostly washes his forearms and his genitals. Several times he tries to leave the shower and I tell him "Not yet." I tug the shower door shut.

When I am done washing and rinsing him I shut the water off and follow him out of the shower. He reaches for the shorts; I take them away and hand him a towel. I grab a towel. He dries some of the front, I dry the rest.

I prompt him to lean against the counter and I help him put on a pair of pull-ups. He then grabs the shorts and puts them on. Sometimes I feel very efficient because I stay bent over and George lifts each foot in turn as I pull the pull-ups over each foot and far enough up his leg that he can pull them up. Then staying bent I reach for the shorts, and he steps into each leg of the shorts. He can still pull them up, button, zip and fasten the belt.

I go into his closet and pull out a shirt and hand it to him. I grab his shoes. I walk to the dresser and pull out a pair of socks. I walk to my closet and put on a robe. I walk to the dining room and pull out a chair and set him in it. I hand him his socks and put the shoes on the floor. I go to the kitchen, pour him a cup of coffee and prepare his bowl of cereal. I set them in front of him.

I go back to the bedroom, remove my robe and climb into the shower to clean myself. After I am dried and dressed except for my shoes I go back in the shower and wipe it down with a micro cloth to keep the grime from building up.

I gather the wet stuff off his bed for the trash and the laundry basket.

I put a load in the washing machine.

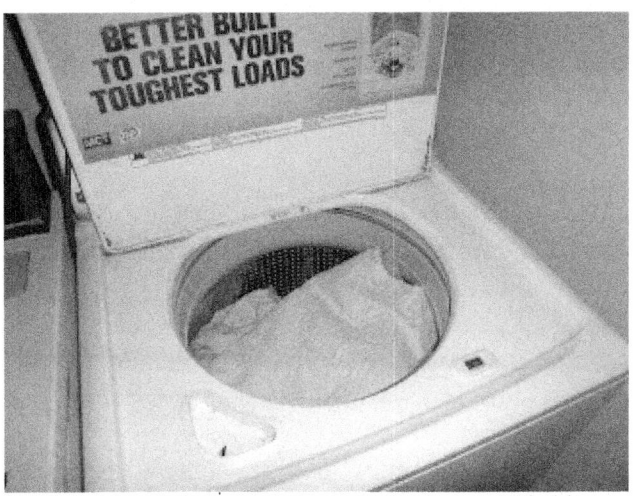

I come back into the house. George is done with his cereal and has placed his dirty, dripping bowl into the dishwasher with the clean dishes. I say nothing. I notice a bulge in the back of his pants.

I say, "Come on, let's get cleaned up." And I go into the bathroom. He follows behind.

I help him remove his shoes and socks and pants and I have him turn around and face the sink. I put on gloves and I clean him up. After each wipe he wants to move to grab his pants. I keep saying, "Not yet."

Cleaned and dressed again I put him in front of the TV and get a movie started for him. He watches cartoons, doggie movies, romances. I think this morning I put on *Paddington Bear*.

I go back in the bathroom, spritz and wipe the counter where he leaned and the floor where flakes of pooh have landed. I tie up the bag in the trash can, remove it, and ready a fresh one.

I walk back out to the curb this time, where I have placed the trash can as it is trash pick-up day.

As George watches *Paddington*, I wash my hands, and make and eat a salad for breakfast. Then I prepare the bikes for riding. I fill the water bottles and put them on the bike. I put my purse, keys and phone on the bike. I gather jackets, hats and gloves because it is nippy out today.

When everything is ready it is 9 a.m. I go get George, bundle him up, and settle him on his trike. I climb onto the front trike of the tandem and I realize I don't have my clip-on bike shoes. I hesitate; worried that George will start to pedal while I am running in to change my shoes.

I get down in front of his face so he can see me well. I tell him twice what I am doing. I urge him not to pedal. I move fast. He is still in place when I return. I sigh with relief.

We bike to Wallace Brooks and smile as we greet other smiling faces in our bike group. As we ride south I struggle to go fast enough but not too fast. Sometimes George pedals, sometimes he doesn't.

We bike about eight miles to Floral City. I help George off the trike and he follows me into the restroom.

I go first and then he stands at the toilet. I rush out to the bike to grab the diaper bag. Back in the restroom George is still standing at the toilet waiting to urinate without success. I know his pull-ups are wet. So while he is standing there I pull down his shorts and his pull-ups. I try to get him to step out of his shorts, but he does not comprehend or he is focused on the task at hand.

I am bent over, hanging onto his shorts, encouraging him to step out. Then I hear it, right next to my ear... poop emerging... and then... PLOP!

"Don't move!" I tell him over and over. I didn't want him to step in it or get his shorts full of it. I reach in the diaper bag and slide on the gloves, all the while telling him, "Don't move!"

I reach out in reaction as I see the next ball of pooh, the size of a lemon, emerging. I catch it.

Uhhh, yeah, I can't believe it. I just caught a ball of gooey pooh and it is now sitting on my gloved hand. I don't know what to think.

What goes through my mind?

"Good catch!" Ha-ha.

George is doing his nervous, teary laugh. I am guessing he comprehends what just happened for just a second.

I drop the ball of pooh into the toilet.

The good news is we got through it without poopy socks or shorts.

When we exited the bathroom our whole group was gone. I put the electric assist up to level two most of the way to get to Nobleton. The group had just ordered when we arrived. We didn't miss the fun.

This morning is *not* every morning. But I often think after a strenuous morning about how grateful I am to be younger and fitter than most caregivers. Can you imagine someone caring for their spouse like this when they are in their 80's and not so physically able? This is physical as well as emotional work.

Still Having Fun

In March and April the snowbirds depart for their northern homes. Before many of them went, I hosted a happy hour and salad bar at our house. We had a good time.

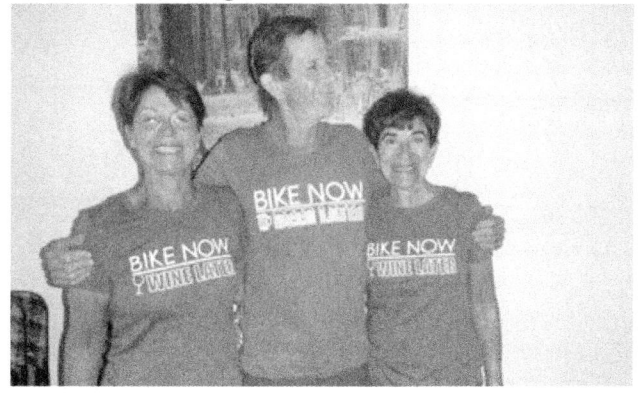

Through Decline, Glimpses of George

May 15, 2018

As I write this, George is watching his third episode in a row of *Top Gear*. It is a program on Amazon Prime about cars. There are three guys, joking around, racing cars, destroying cars, and having fun doing it. I ask George how he is doing and he chuckles.

Watching hours of programs about machines is just the kind of thing the old George would have done. He used to spend hours watching *How It's Made*. Finding this interest for him is like having respite. I can work in the garden, chat with the neighbors, or make phone calls and he is content.

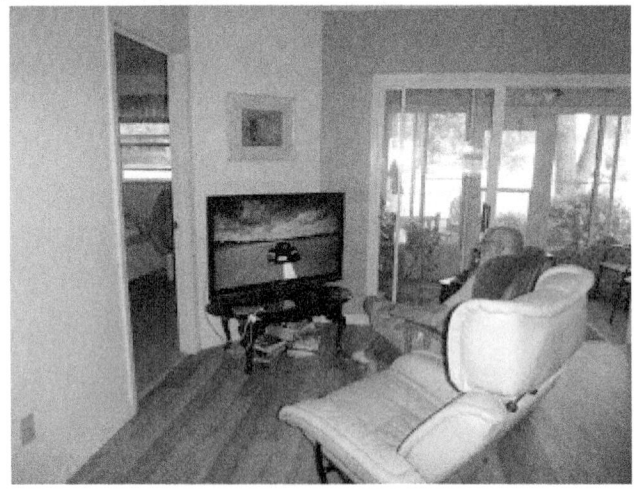

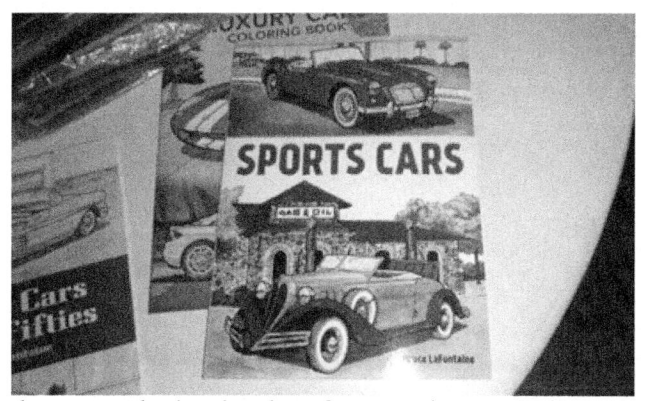

I ordered some coloring books of cars. Those are the ones he will still color. He is not very interested in coloring in any of the other books anymore.

I have set up my computer on a card table on the porch so I can see him as he watches TV. When he needs to get up or when the movie stops playing he doesn't call for me. He makes no sound at all. He just looks for me and struggles to get up. Once when I was on the computer in the den I stepped out to check on him and I found him on the floor by his chair. No grunt, no yell, no banging, no sounds....

He is getting more unsteady on his feet. Sometimes when I take him for a walk we go part way down the block and then I turn us around because already he is walking into the curb, or leaning too far forward causing him to do a stiff-legged run. The Divas now have some equipment to loan out due to the death of some of our "princes." I borrowed a transport chair and now I take it with me to stores and on walks, just in case. He sits in it easily and knows to put down the foot pads and rest his feet on the foot pads.

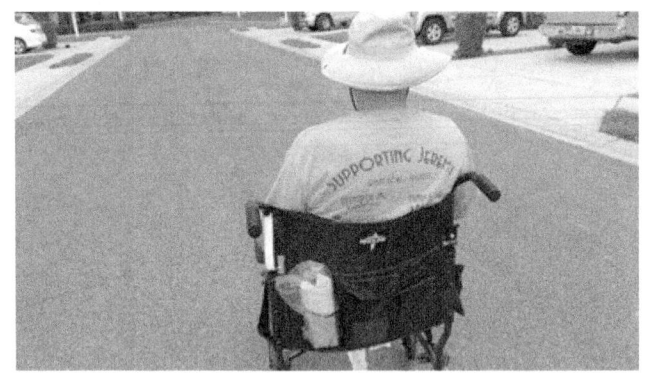

Our friend Debra suggested I get a disabled parking space permit prescription from his doctor. I suppose it is time.

Though on a good day, with some rests to get him to correct his posture and balance, he can walk the four blocks to the clubhouse and back.

I wonder if he is depressed. Does this make him sad or is he too foggy to think about it at all? I want to ask him, but I know that is too deep a topic for him to comprehend. Is he lonely not being able to talk? He still seems to enjoy the company of our bike friends and others.

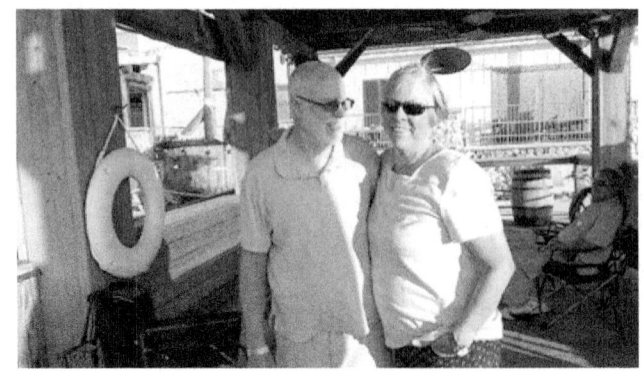

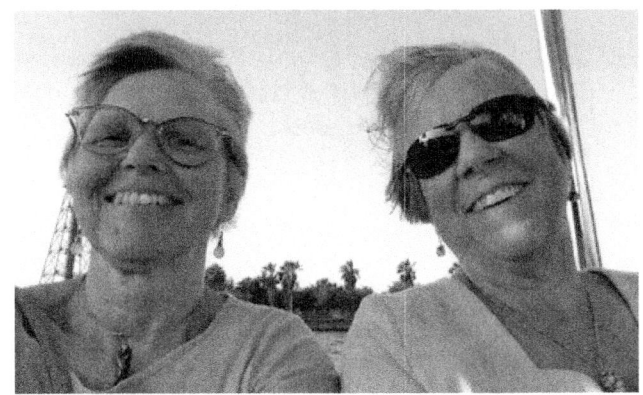

I am now working to gather pictures of his younger years. I am trying to remember who he was. Even I, who spent so many years with him, am forgetting. It seems to me I like him better now. Quiet, compliant... gosh, that is a terrible thing to say! Certainly I miss being able to share my day with him, to talk about people and places and dreams and events.

Parts of him are still here. He still sometimes will close a drawer or turn off a light after me. He still removes his shirt in the same way so it remains right-side-out. He still smiles at people. When he hugs me he pats my bottom and then tries to get his hands into my back pockets. I soak in those hugs. I know I will miss them when they are gone.

We are triking still. And the other day we went to The Villages with Debra and Glen and took a quick boat ride. I want to do more boat rides. I think George enjoyed it and so did the rest of us.

On Friday last week Glen came and stayed with George until the bus came to take George to the Key. Debra and Trudy and I left early to go to Silver Springs for a day of kayaking.

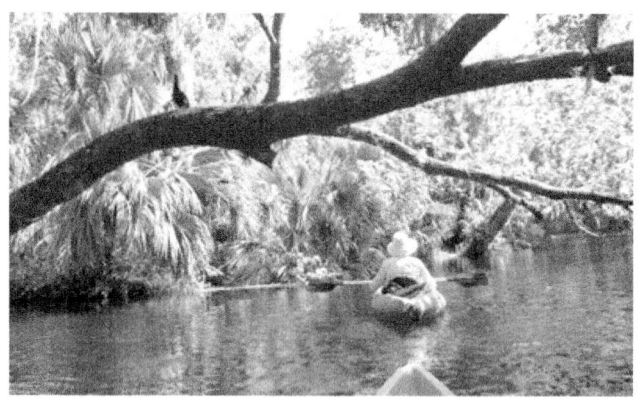

I am looking into a boat ride from Yankeetown. I have heard good things about it.

Oh! Before I leave, I wanted to let you know I have rented out the second room. Now both bedrooms are rented to guys who are working third shift on the new Duke Energy gas plant in Crystal River. The new guy moved in on Monday and tells me he left his wallet in Houston, TX. He has his mom sending it express. Next time I post to this blog I will have an update on that saga. I am not worried yet. He calls me "Ma'am." He says, "Yes, Ma'am."

Falling Forward

Wednesday, May 16, 2018

Witness to a Fall

George fell yesterday. I was gathering stuff up to head over to the clubhouse for happy hour. I mentioned where we were going to George, and out the door he went. He usually goes to the first car he comes to and waits at the passenger door with his hand on the handle.

I rushed to gather stuff and get his transport chair (wheelchair) out of the garage. Then I am heading down the drive, and I see he is up to the corner already, half a block away. He knows where we are going and he is moving fast.

He leans forward when he walks, and stopping is hard for him. I yell at him to slow down. I tell him to stop. He tries; he always turns his whole body to look at me, and then he is falling sideways so he has to keep going straight. "Put weight on your heels," I holler.

He walks almost a whole block more - with me telling him to move onto the grass because I know he is going to fall, but I can't get there fast enough. He moves onto the grass but then heads back toward the street and he makes a belly flop onto the thin strip of grass between the sidewalk and the street. He didn't catch himself at all.

I lie next to him on my belly and check him out. Then I show him how to get up on his hands and knees. Two neighbors stop to offer help. I refuse, but one comes over and offers George a hand and George gets up fine. I put him in the chair. He has a scratch on his face and hand. It could have been a lot worse. He was OK; I had a nice time at the happy hour.

Spiffing Up My Old Trike

When Glen and Debra suggested I get my old trike painted, I at first hesitated. Then they investigated and found a place that does powder coat painting and it will only cost me $200. Again I hesitated.

Then Glen offered to disassemble my trike so all I had to do was deliver the frame to the painter which is within two miles of our house.

I stop into the painter and find a lovely light purple to match the flowery painted fenders I have.

Years ago when George got his trike custom painted, he helped me find a painter to paint my fenders. His custom paint job cost over a thousand dollars. Mine cost me $150 dollars. I love my fenders with purple and yellow flowers, teal and orange butterflies, and shimmery dragon-flies. They are beautiful.

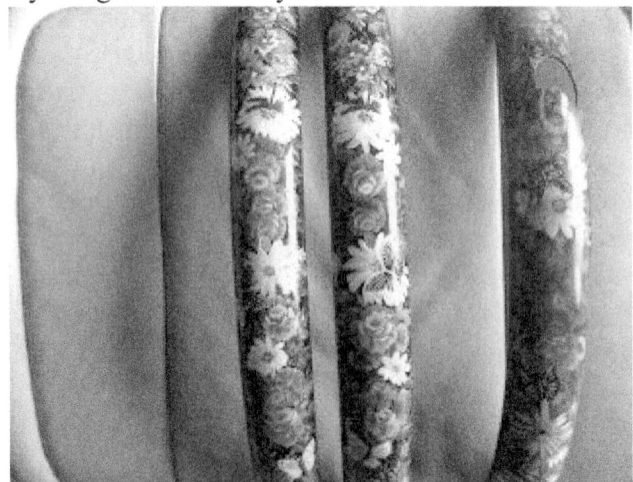

Thanks to Glen and Debra for their encouragement and for the tedious task of taking my trike apart. Glen has ordered some new gears for me and I am getting excited.

Don't I have the most awesome friends???

I bought a new trunk and I am getting that and a helmet painted too.

My friend Karon, who is artsy and creative, is going to help me figure out a way to "enhance" my helmet with some decorative sun protections. A wine and creativity night coming soon - Wowza!

My Dementia Diva friends Karon and Dianne both have lost their spouses this year.

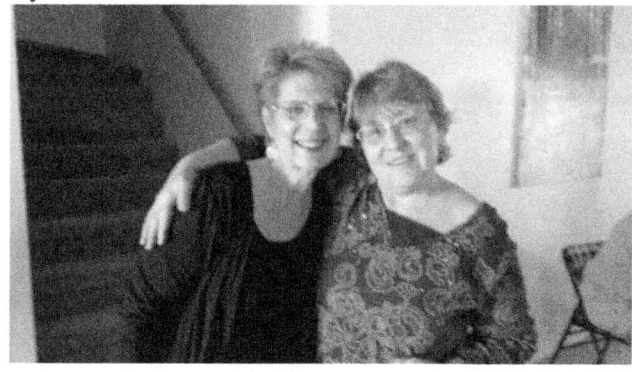

Renter Update, Warm Showers

Renter Update

I thought you would want to know what happened with the renter who arrived on Monday but said, "I left my wallet in Texas," and could not pay rent yet. On Thursday when we got home he was gone already. I put a note and an empty envelope in his room and said he was to put the money in the envelope and slide it under the den door on Friday or he could move his stuff out and hand in the key.

I called our handyman and he said it was about $375 to change two doors to combination locks.

On Friday morning when I checked my phone there were five text messages from the renter (Daniel) with explanations, excuses, sad-face emoji's. I did not text him back.

At noon I checked the mail thinking there might be something there from his mom. There was nothing. I texted Daniel.

A bit later I get a response in a voice mail. She is not sending the wallet. But he is going to get money wired from his bank (wow, why didn't he do that earlier?) and he was going out right now to get some money and bring it back.

George was at Key all day Friday. I went into the den and locked the door feeling no need to interact with the renter without getting money first. (I didn't want to deal with any challenges to my decision to oust him.) Besides, I had Personal Fitness Trainer video-lessons in anatomy to watch.

I heard the renter return and then later slide an envelope under the door. A note of apology, rent, and about $160 toward June's rent. YEAH!!!! I typed out a statement stating the amount due on May 31st.

Alzheimer's Symptoms

An obsession with leaves....

Did I tell you that the other day (about a month ago) we were dining outside at the picnic table and after George was done with his salad he began to pick up the dead leaves that were stuck between the slates of the table and eat them? He would make a face like it tasted terrible, but then fish out another one and put it in his mouth. The only way to stop him was to move him away from the table.

Leaning right....

For more than a year George has been leaning when I take him on walks.

This past week Debra and Glen had us over for dinner. During dinner George was leaning to his right... collapsing right? I would straighten him out and immediately he would lean again. As a caregiver we learn to relax about these things. It is what it is, I can persist and get upset or I can just let it be.

Later I put him on Glen and Debra's couch in front of a movie. We dead-locked the front door, took the key with us and went out on the back porch with a glass of wine. YES!

Later when I checked on him he was leaning way to the right and his shirt was all wet where he had been drooling. Oh my!

Breathing Interruptions....

Early on in the illness George started snoring more and would... get stuck and not breathe. It would drive me nuts because I was always waiting for him to take a breath. Other than his jerking, it was one of the main reasons I moved to sleeping in a different room. I just couldn't sleep in the same room, and I really needed to sleep in order to care for him and run our household.

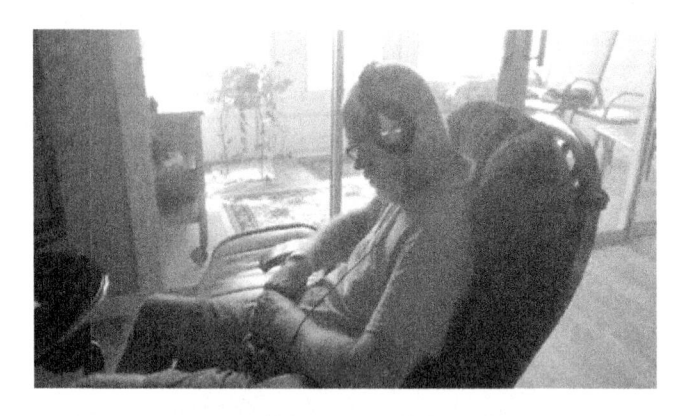

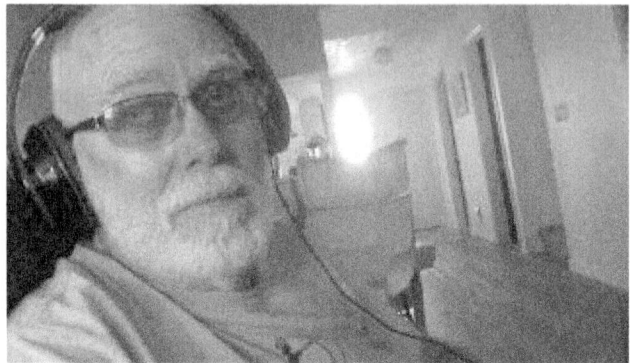

Lately I have caught him snoring in his chair. Some people with sleep apnea sleep in a chair. George didn't ever snore in a seated position. Now, he sleeps more when I set him in front of the TV, and a few times I have heard him snore and get stuck, then gasp, snore and get stuck. I have tried waking him to stop it, but then a few minutes later, there he is, nodding off, stopping and starting. It is what it is.

Right now I am in the patio, my laptop on a card-table. I have closed the patio door and turned on the ceiling fan so I don't have to hear it.

OH NO!!!! DIARRHEA!

OMG! Just when I think I am all used to cleaning George's bottom....

This Thursday we were biking south with the group. It was great and fun. We were ahead of many in the group, so I knew we had time to stop in Floral City at the bathroom. I took the diaper bag into the bathroom with us. Just like a girl scout, or is it a boy scout. Always prepared... just in case.

George unzips his pants and starts walking to the toilet pulling the front of his pull-up down, getting ready to stand and pee in the toilet. Only what I see is gooey smelly pooh all over his pubic hair, penis and testicles.

Yikes! I try to get the gloves on while trying to keep him from putting his fingers into the pooh.

OK, no more details. Suffice it to say he was obsessed with touching it and could not follow commands. I had a hard time getting him to lift his feet out of his pants. I ended up removing his shirt because he was touching it. Oh my.

I went through a whole container of wet wipes even with using toilet paper and rinsing some of the wet wipes. I could not get him clean. So I did the best we could, cleaned up the bathroom, and then we rode home to shower.

I remember my Wisconsin bike-friend whose husband had Alzheimer's. Her first experience with his incontinence was in a store bathroom and he had diarrhea. OH MY! Now I know what she was talking about. What a *MESS*!

Trike Painted

It is beautiful! I am so happy with it!

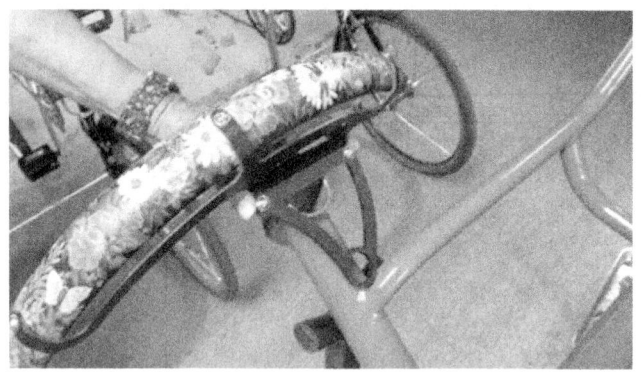

The trunk and the helmet aren't painted yet. They are plastic and went to a different painter.

Glen is now enjoying the joys and frustrations of re-assembling my trike. I told him to keep a tally of parts and tools he purchases to complete the job so I can reimburse him. It really is unbelievable how fortunate and blessed I am to be surrounded by such great and supportive friends.

This Week

It has been a rainy week. This week we had our first Warmshowers guest in a long time. A couple who lives in Lady Lake, Florida, came to stay one night. I told them I had both guestrooms rented out but they were welcome to stay on our screened porch. They were grateful to be out of the rain and rode 60 miles, much of it through a downpour, to get to our house.

They were very sweet to George. Steve would get down at eye-level and talk directly to George. George began to respond a bit (mostly with head nods and his teary-laugh). I told them they were welcome to stop again on their return trip. Steve and Nancy offered to help me out with tasks or George sitting. You can meet the nicest people through Warmshowers!

Last night we dined out with bike friends. It was fun and so nice to still be invited to these gatherings.

I ordered George pasta and the long noodles kept him busy during the hour I was able to stay and visit.

Even with George's decline we were able to bike today on the tandem trike.

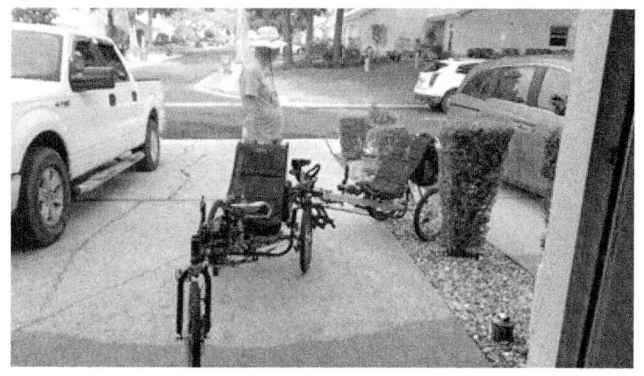

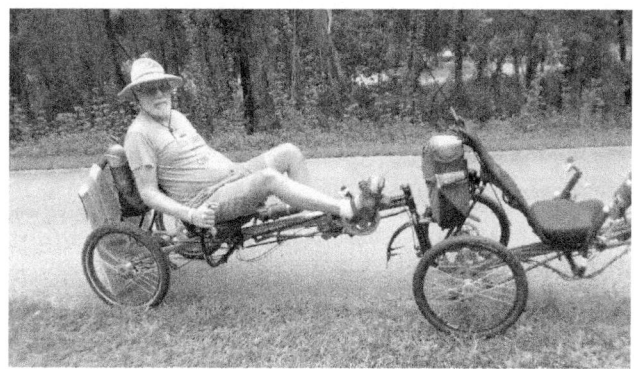

Now George is once again sitting in front of *The Boss Baby* movie, sleeping and snoring and drooling. Still loving him! Life is a trip!

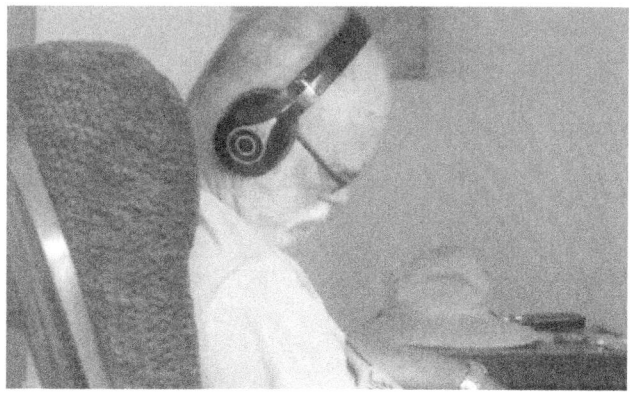

My Sweet George, Gone Too Soon

May 20, 2018

Last night George was even more wobbly on his feet. I was afraid I would not be able to get him in bed if I didn't take him in early. He was in bed by seven.

When I went to check on him later he was kneeling on the floor with his face on the bed. He was so weak I could not move him. I leaned over him and kissed his back and said, "I love you *sooo* much." and I felt him relax.

I enlisted Tirso's help (the guy renting the upstairs bedroom). We got him in bed OK. When I checked on him later he was breathing and in bed.

In the morning I went to get him up at 7 a.m. and he was on his back on the floor. I could not get him up. So I covered him to keep him warm and called my friend Debra.

Debra came and sat with me. George had a Do NOT RESUSCITATE order. I wanted to honor it. I didn't want to send him to the hospital.

After Debra and I had breakfast I checked on him again and he wasn't breathing. He was gone, just like that.

Sweet George.

What do you do first when something like this happens?

I called 911. I had learned through the Divas and through the Neptune Society where I had made George's pre-arrangements for cremation that I was required to call 911 when he died. I told the operator he was gone, and he had a DNR and it wasn't an emergency.

The paramedics came and pulled out their box with wires. I thought they were going to try to start up his heart again, but they assured me and Debra they were putting wires on him to make sure he was dead.

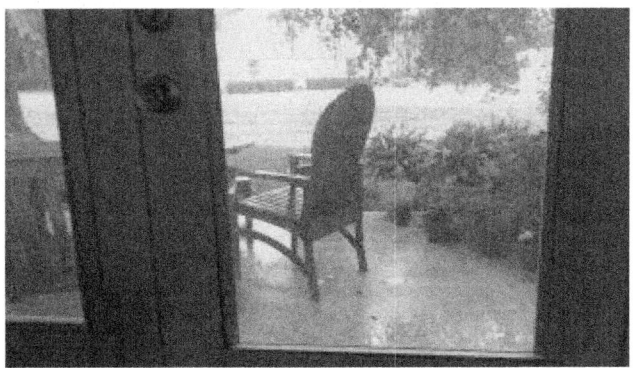

I called my next-door neighbors, Mari and Jerry, and they came over to sit with me on the porch while I went through this horrible period of waiting for them to take care of the legalities of getting George's doctor on the phone to agree to sign the death certificate.

My heart was/is breaking. It helped to have these great friends there also shedding tears for my lovely George. His smile and good nature in his dementia years were fun and enjoyable. Many had learned to love his sweet nature.

When the ambulance left, we had to wait for the Neptune Society to arrive. A sheriff's deputy remained to wait for the hearse also. My friends took me next door, and Glen stayed to help if needed getting George's body into the hearse.

It was after noon by the time they pulled away with George's body, and I said another goodbye.

Our last day together was good. We went to the Hen House for breakfast and dined with our bike friends. We biked south until the promise of rain chased us north. George watched TV. It was raining; he kept getting up and walking out the front door.

I tried to distract him and I turned on some music. We danced together some fast and slow dances with a CD that Frankie had given me. You know when I say dance, I mean George stood and I moved, right?

He gave me this picture he colored at the Key Center. "I did this," he told me several times.

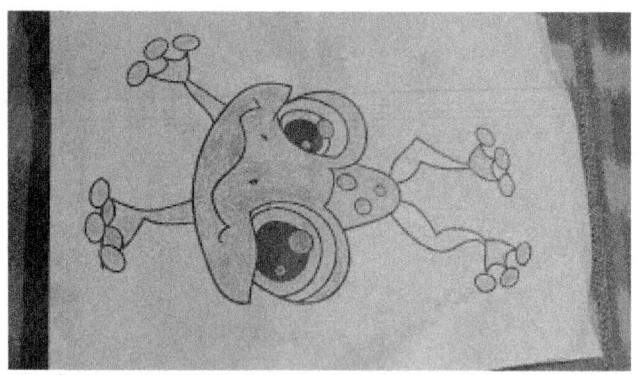

It seems he left too soon.

Just this week I was wondering how much longer I would have the strength to lift him up out of a chair.

I am sad, yet I am not sad. My heart breaks and it is filled with joy for the moments we had.

After George's body was taken away, I followed Debra and Glen home and spent the afternoon on their porch making calls and crying.

Then Debra and Glen joined me with wine and enchiladas and memories. We were actually laughing!

Friends, Family, Therapy, and Sleep-overs

May 27, 2018

I have been getting messages from readers of this blog asking me how to find out how I am doing. So consider this a postscript.... There may be a few.

Each person who goes through the death of a beloved spouse, I suppose, experiences it differently.

I know that my heart hurts. My intestines are protesting from the stress of loss and change. I can think I am moving smoothly and then break down in tears.

I am one of the fortunate ones.

Surrounded by friends and following a year or two of learning to accept offers of help, I have been dining with friends once or twice a day every day, alone just enough to process a little at a time. I am taking this loss in small bites.

My sister Mary has been there to accept my calls and to check in with me, my stepdaughter Jodie and I have talked several times this first week, and I have called and gotten comforting calls from my son Jeremy. I have gotten calls from friends in Wisconsin and Canada.

Debra has offered a bed in her home for the week that I have gratefully taken advantage of after one horrible night of anxious insomnia at home. I keep my pillows and my blanket in my car for now. Not ready just yet to try to face the thoughts of how I could have done better or differently in his last hours.

I stepped right back into routine on Monday (George passed on Sunday). I felt out of body, yet very much experiencing the pain of my broken heart. I reached out for hugs and I got them.

Wednesday the cards started coming in the mailbox.

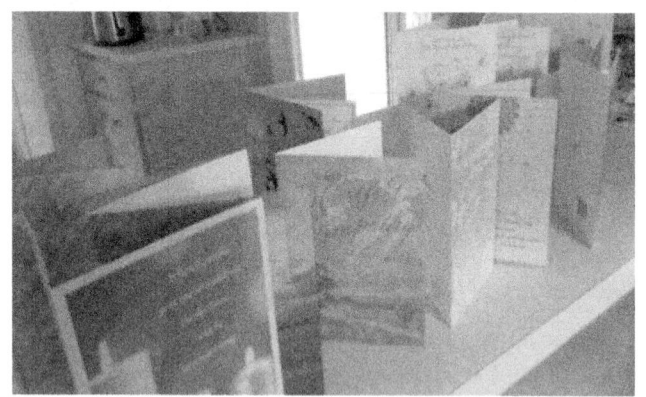

What I love reading are memories of a time before George's illness. So much of those memories have faded. I will post later, memories of George.

Monday I even drove to Memory Lane.

Memory Lane hugs were especially comforting. Dianne and Karon were there, recently widowed themselves due in part to Alzheimer's disease or dementia. Dianne and Karon both offered for me to spend a night in their guest beds. Paul set up a time to feed the three of us at his house, cooking us a meal all while caring for his sweet wife. He is an Amazing Prince. Karon invited me to come to her home and dine with her friends who were gathering for supper on Friday. Such wonderful support from my support group family!

Another friend, who lost her husband almost two years ago, called and offered advice and I got the name of her therapist and set up an appointment. It's this Tuesday already!

Yesterday was Saturday. I went to breakfast with the bike group. Rode a bit then returned to the Hen House for breakfast with the Dementia Divas and Princes. I rode some more and then when I pulled into my neighborhood I saw Debra and Glen leaving. They had finished assembling my newly painted trike!!!

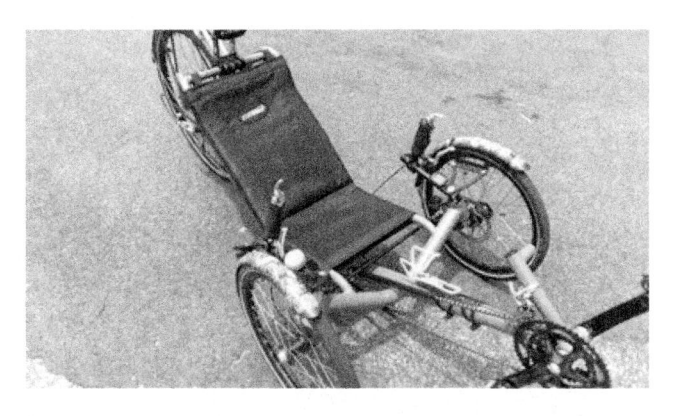

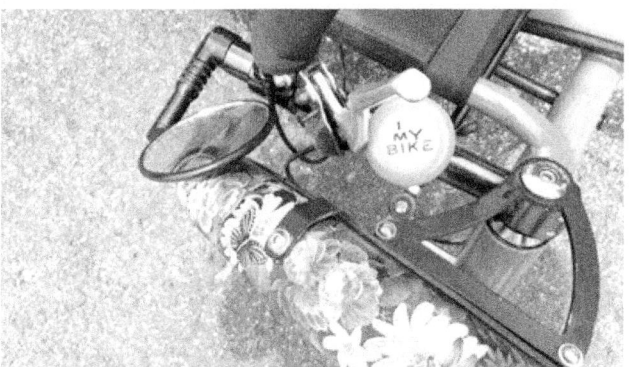

I took it only 1/2 a block and it started to rain and I started to sob. George would have been so happy for me. I am happy for me. It runs so beautifully, new gears, new chain, cleaned up, and totally awesome in every way. THANK YOU, GLEN!! (And thank you, Debra, for labeling all the parts and helping him along the way.) LOVE YOU GUYS!!

May I learn to be as good a friend as the friends I have around me.

There is a tropical storm in the Gulf and it is sending lots of rain over us here. When I can get out for a walk, my footsteps are not fast. I had yearned to walk *fast*. Now the energy is gone. I know it will return.

So much of George is in me, with me. He taught me patience. He believed in my intelligence back when I did not. He believed in my ability to learn. He showed me how to live with integrity. He taught me how to love.

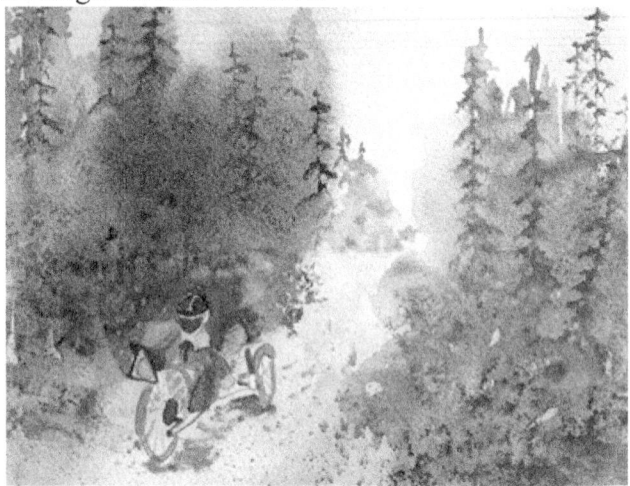

George painted the picture above during our search for a diagnosis. He was under the instruction of Jude Caborn, an artist neighbor at the time. He gave up painting after this one great picture.

THANK YOU to all who have reached out to me and/or sent me prayers or good energy. It is so helpful.

The Essence of George...

June 2, 2018

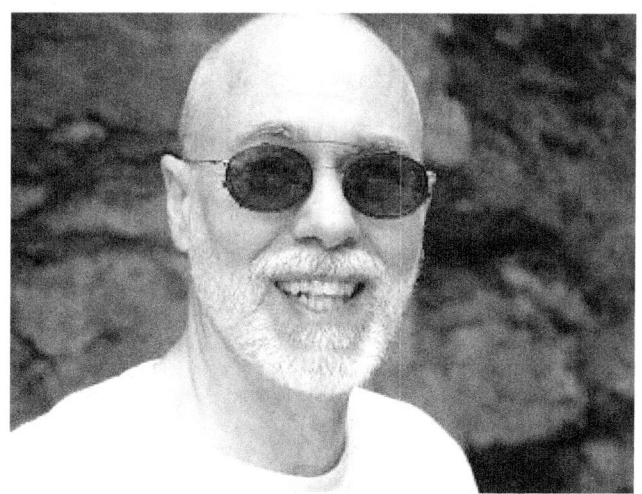

In the past couple years I have had a difficult time recalling who George was before dementia. I have tried and only could remember the parts that angered me. Maybe that is why it was so easy to love him so much as he lived with dementia. I have heard similar reports from other dementia caregiver widows.

After his passing I started to look for those memories in pictures and in stories told.

Of course, George had a life before me. But that was over 41 years ago!

He was the oldest of five children.

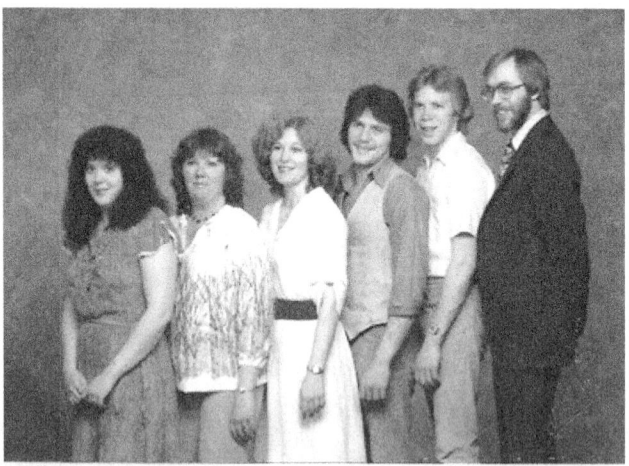

He joined the navy at 17 and served on an aircraft carrier.

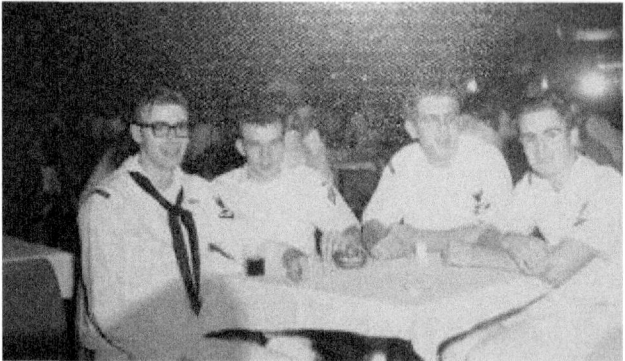

This comment was sent to my brother-in-law Dave who used to work at the same place as George before I even met George. A fellow co-worker commented:

...When I first hired on at RMG back in 1976, Guthrie held George in high esteem and called him a "crackerjack" designer.

He had a very artistic and beautiful flow to his drawings, and they were very artful as well as good engineering drawings.

I remember studying how he drew stuff, and copying the way he used line weights to distinguish between different parts of the drawing.

His printing was very stylized and impressive. I remember he did an illustration for RMG of an operator feeding the wire into a header with ease because of the wire relaxer roller.

"An RMG Exclusive!"

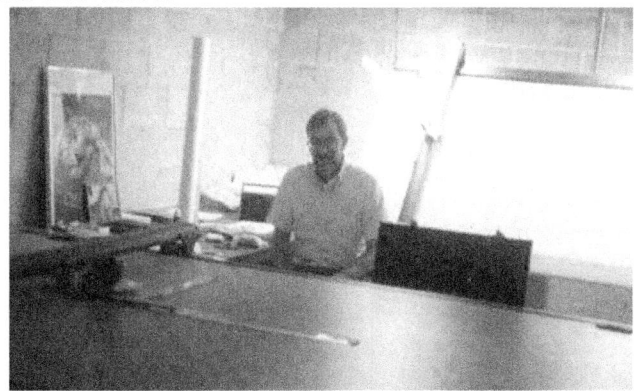

After his design services moved from pencil and paper drawings to computer-generated drawings printed with ink, he changed the name of his business from Straley's Services to Rentapen, Inc.

Oh what a gift, to have that memory of his neat drawing and printing brought back vividly. He was so disciplined in his work. I was a free spirit and he was so regimented. We balanced each other out. He taught me so much!

This memory helps me remember the huge callous he had on his finger from holding those drawing pencils tight. That leads to memories of just sitting and holding hands... nice....

George was a very hard worker. He worked full time and went to school full time earning three Associate Degrees... Mechanical Drawing, Electronics, Computer Science. He started his business the year we got married.

He was an innovator. When the first affordable home computers came out - Commodore 64, remember? - he purchased one and spent hours after work programming it and then playing the "Pong" game he had programmed.

After he purchased his first 2D computer-aided drafting program (CAD) for the business, George immediately went to work to make it more efficient to use. Together with his engineers he created a colorful tablet overlay and programed the tablet to get to functions with just one or two clicks. Then he spent hours plotting and coloring and laminating the tablets to sell to other engineers.

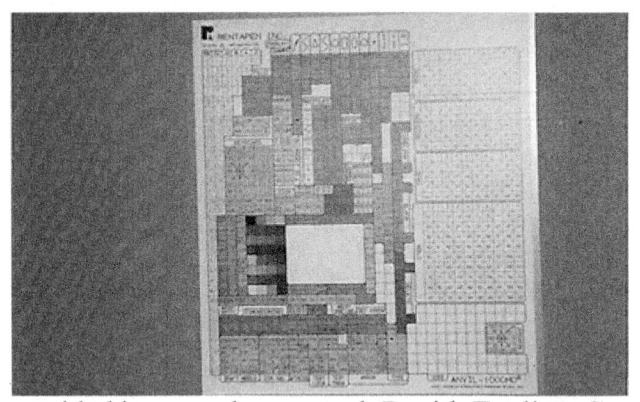

Together with his team he created Rapid Tooling Components that are still used in the machine tool industry to fine-tune the location of production parts in a manufacturing machine.

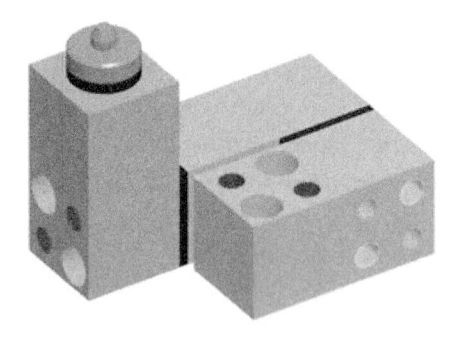

He worked hard to grow and maintain his Mechanical Design business... Rentapen. It was a tough business which rode the highs and lows on the economic booms and busts of the country. The most employees Rentapen ever had was 14, and the least was... well, just George. He would not give up. He kept searching for answers, taking courses, listening to educational and motivational tapes.

George loved my parents as if they were his own. He never complained about weekend hours spent hanging out with them.

He blended into our family. My brother once thanked George. He said George's support had made me a better person.

My favorite picture of us isn't because it flatters us – we are both in sweat pants. We had helped my brother-in-law Dave and my sister Mary cut down a tree. Afterward George set up the timer on his camera to get a picture of us sitting on the downed tree. He ran back to the log and went to sit down but overshot and landed on his back, feet in air. We managed to get him back up before the camera went off. Mary and Dave, George and I all laughing. A great moment.

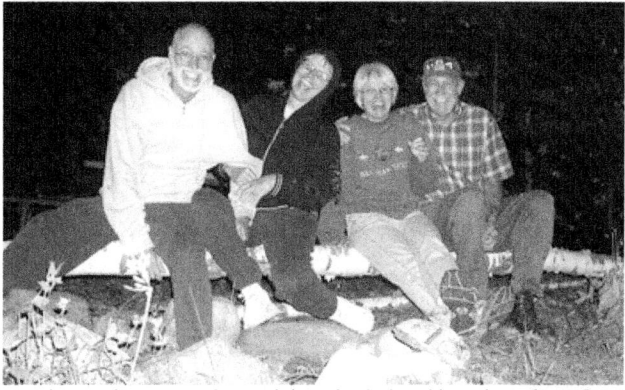

And below is a picture of our blended family shortly after we got married in 1976.

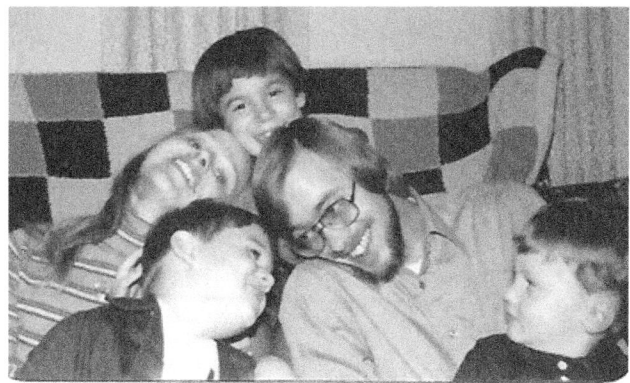

He hiked with me and biked with me and trusted me. Even in his demented state he never doubted that what I was doing was for his good. I was and *am* incredibly blessed. As we grew older he was most proud of our long marriage. He told me he loved me *every day*. I don't know when that started, but once it did it went on well over 20 years and into his dementia years.

When we were working we enjoyed weekend bike adventures with our Wisconsin bike friends.

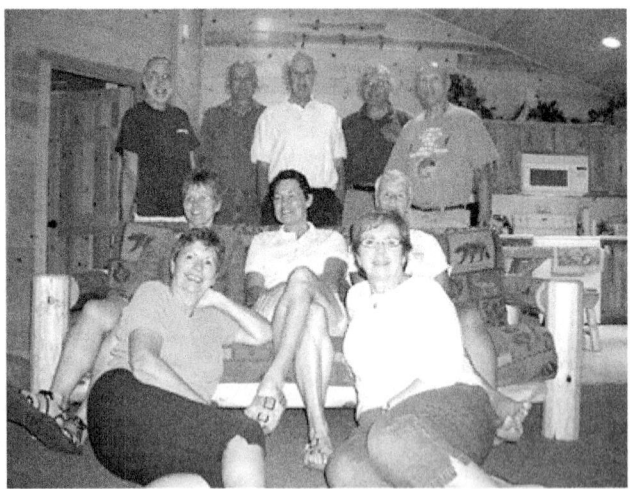

He biked around Wisconsin with me in 2008.

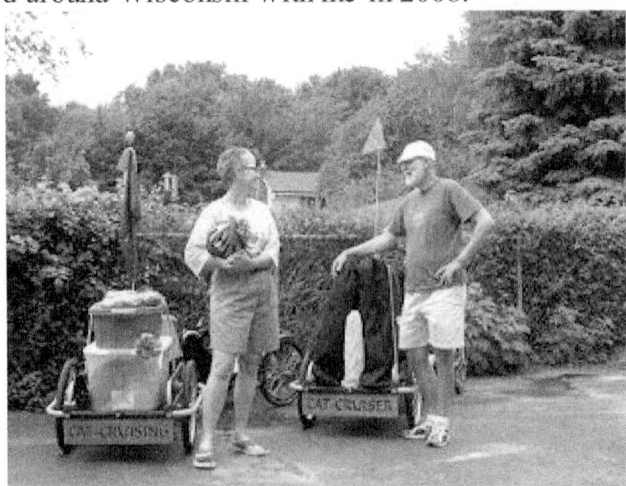

He biked from Illinois to Florida with me even in his early days of dementia, before he knew he had it, before his diagnosis.

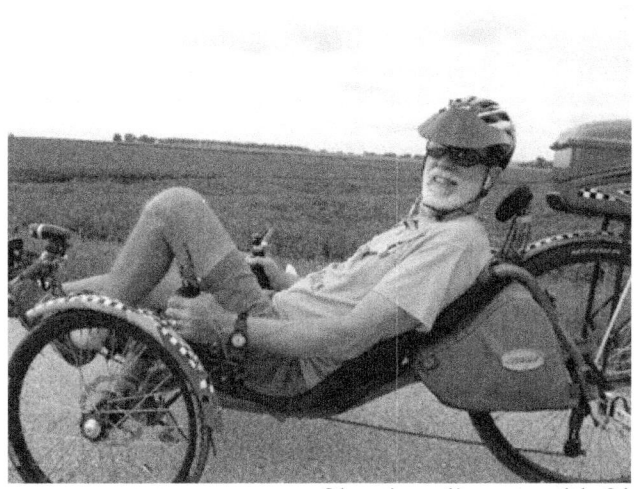

Together we were a super team of hosting dinners with friends and hosting bike tourists as they pedaled their way through the area (via Warmshowers.org).

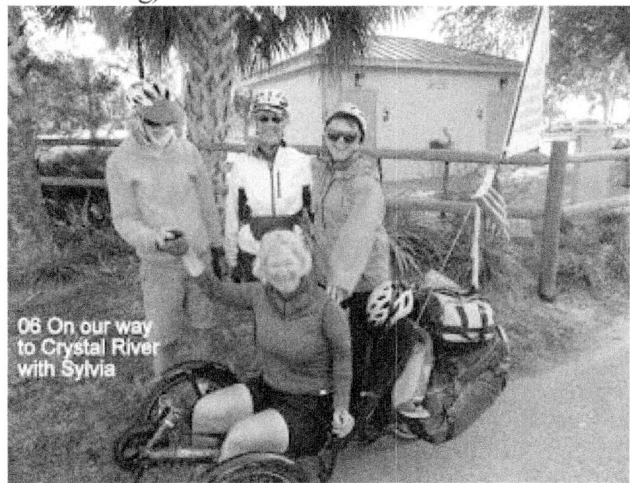

06 On our way to Crystal River with Sylvia

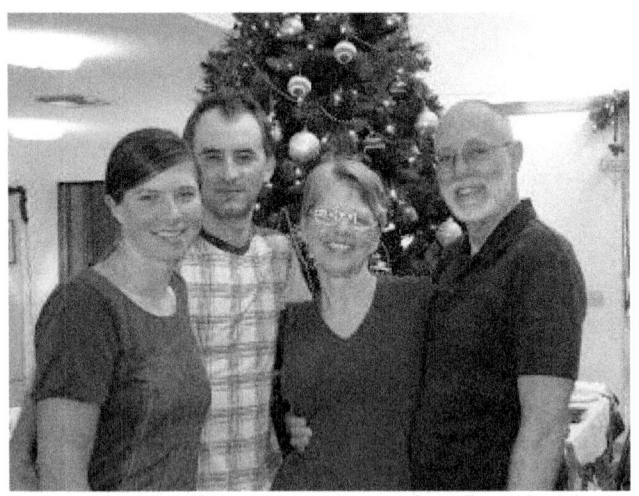

In the 70's and 80's he was among the first in the recycling movement! Before it was generally popular we were recycling and when we would have our "Grub Clubs" with our group of friends in Wisconsin he would harass our hosts and guests if they did not recycle. He spoke out at stores when they wanted to bag one item. "If I can carry it to the register in my hands I can carry it to the car in my hands," he would say.

He made it a point to use people's names. In the checkout line or the restaurant or anywhere, he would learn the server's name and use it often. That was another thing I loved about him.

A person's whole essence, their life, cannot be fully documented or honored in a few stories and pictures.

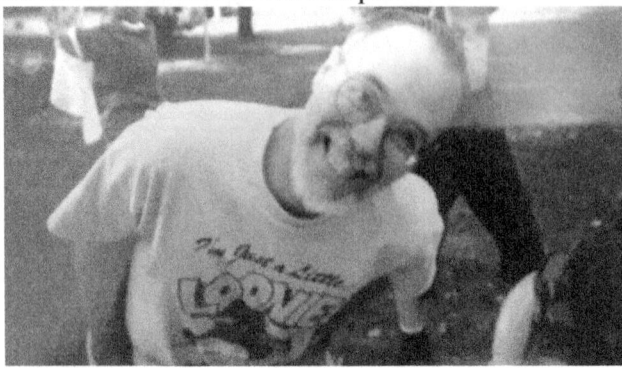

This attempt to find the memory of who George was leaves me loving him again the way he was before dementia....

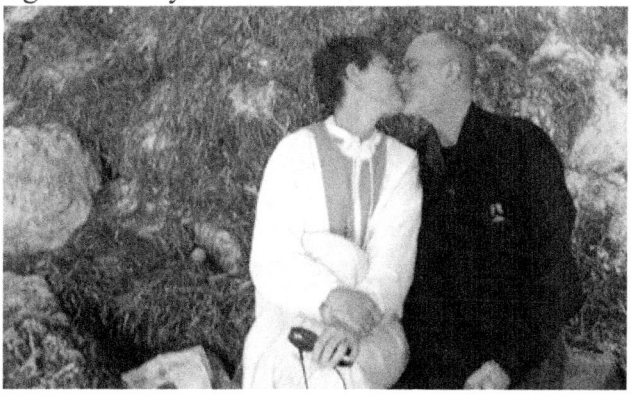

"The George" tandem has been donated to the Withlacoochee Bicycle Riders group. It will continue to provide riding pleasure to Withlacoochee Riders as the need arises due to disability. Thanks to the generosity of all those who loved George and made it happen.

To leave a review on Amazon and Goodreads, click on the yellow stars. Share your experience with this book on your social media so that others can find it.

There is lots of Trippin' yet to do. Go to www.susanstraley.com and click JOIN to get on the virtual bus. *Susan*

Resources

The following resources are in no particular order. These are just some of the sources of information we used on our journey.

Elder Options is the state-designated area agency on aging (AAA), Aging & Disability Resource Center (ADRC). Elder Options is charged with administering state and federal grant-funded programs and providing direct services in a 16-county Planning and Service Area (PSA) in North Central Florida, which includes the following counties: Alachua, Bradford, Citrus, Columbia, Dixie, Gilchrist, Hamilton, Hernando, Lafayette, Lake, Levy, Marion, Putnam, Sumter, Suwannee, and Union. Inquire here about the **SAVVY Caregiver training**. It is an excellent class for dementia caregivers. SAVVY Caregiving is also available in an online version for download. www.agingresources.org Phone: 800-963-5337

Alzheimer's Association is the leading voluntary health organization in Alzheimer's care, support and research. www.Alz.org Phone: 800.272.3900

Coping with Dementia is based in Citrus County Florida. Its mission is to make life better for individuals and families living with dementia. Debbie Selsavage leads the organization and was trained by Teepa Snow. She trains service business staff, runs support groups, and educates the public. Phone: 352-422-3663

AARP is a nonprofit, nonpartisan organization that empowers people to choose how they live as they age. It has web pages and booklets proving caregiver support. Phone: 888-687-2277

Alzheimer's Family Organization (AFO) is based in Citrus County, Florida. This organization focuses on helping caregivers have a better quality of life. Visit their helpful links page for all kinds of caregiver resources. www.alzheimersfamily.org Phone: 352-616-0170

Positive Approach to Care was founded by Teepa Snow. It is one of the leading educators on dementia and the care that accompanies it. Teepa Snow has a YouTube channel with educational videos. I especially like her ability to calm an agitated or afraid person with dementia. www.teepasnow.com Phone: 877-877-1671

Memory Lane is the support group we attended every week that we could. It is located at the First Methodist Church in Homosassa, FL. A group of wonderful volunteers kept George and the others occupied while we caregivers met. www.1umc.org/ministry   Phone: 352 628-4083

The Hen House restaurant is the first Certified Dementia Friendly service business in Citrus County, FL. Open for breakfast and lunch and is located at 206 Tompkins St., Inverness, Florida. Phone: 352-419-7942

Greenspeed-trikes is where you can find a list of dealers for the kind of trikes we hooked together to make a tandem. Greenspeed-Trikes.com The USA distributor is located in Illinois. Phone: 618-514-3955

The Hostel Shoppe is a bike shop specializing in recumbent bikes and trikes. This is where I ordered the Greenspeed Anura, the front half of our tandem trike. It is located in Stevens Point, WI. Phone: 800-233-4340

Trailside Bike is a bike shop specializing in recumbent bikes and trikes. This is where they did all the repairs on our tandem trike. It is located in Floral City, FL. Phone: 352-419-4809

Bafang is the type of electric motor that we used on the front trike of the tandem. The USA distributor is at www.BafangUSAdirect.com. Phone: 800-223-0221

Find-M'Friends is based in Citrus County, Florida. It trains bloodhounds to find lost persons. They distribute the scent kits for storing your loved one's scent. Findmfriends.com Phone: 352-613-3486

Catrike is the brand of tricycle that George and I rode for many years. I still ride my purple Expedition model. You will find a list of dealers on their website. www.catrike.com

About the Author

Susan Straley was born with an urge to wander. "My parents were often searching for me. At three years old they found me several blocks away playing in a mud puddle," said Straley.

Straley started to journal at age 16. She began blogging about their travels by trike on Crazyguyonabike.com in 2008. The journal with details and humor quickly gained a following.

Susan Straley lives and bikes in Inverness, Florida.

Susan's first book, *Alzheimer's Trippin' with George: Diagnosis to Discovery in 10,000 Miles* is out in paperback, ebook and audio book.

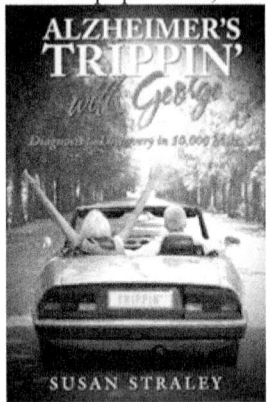

What would you do if you learned that your spouse or partner has progressive dementia, possibly Alzheimer's disease?

This is the brutally honest journal of one spouse and reluctant caregiver that "ran for the hills." Of course she took her husband George along.

What challenges did Susan encounter? How can she enjoy the present — a journey across the U.S.A. - while worrying about the future? How do she and George deal with his increasing dementia symptoms?

And the biggest question of all, after 40 years together, can they remain married and loving through it all?

Travel the U.S.A. along with George. Don't let the number of pages scare you, there are LOTS of pictures. You will glide through the days as they did. You will learn, you will laugh and maybe shed a tear as you too go <u>*Alzheimer's Trippin' with George.*</u>

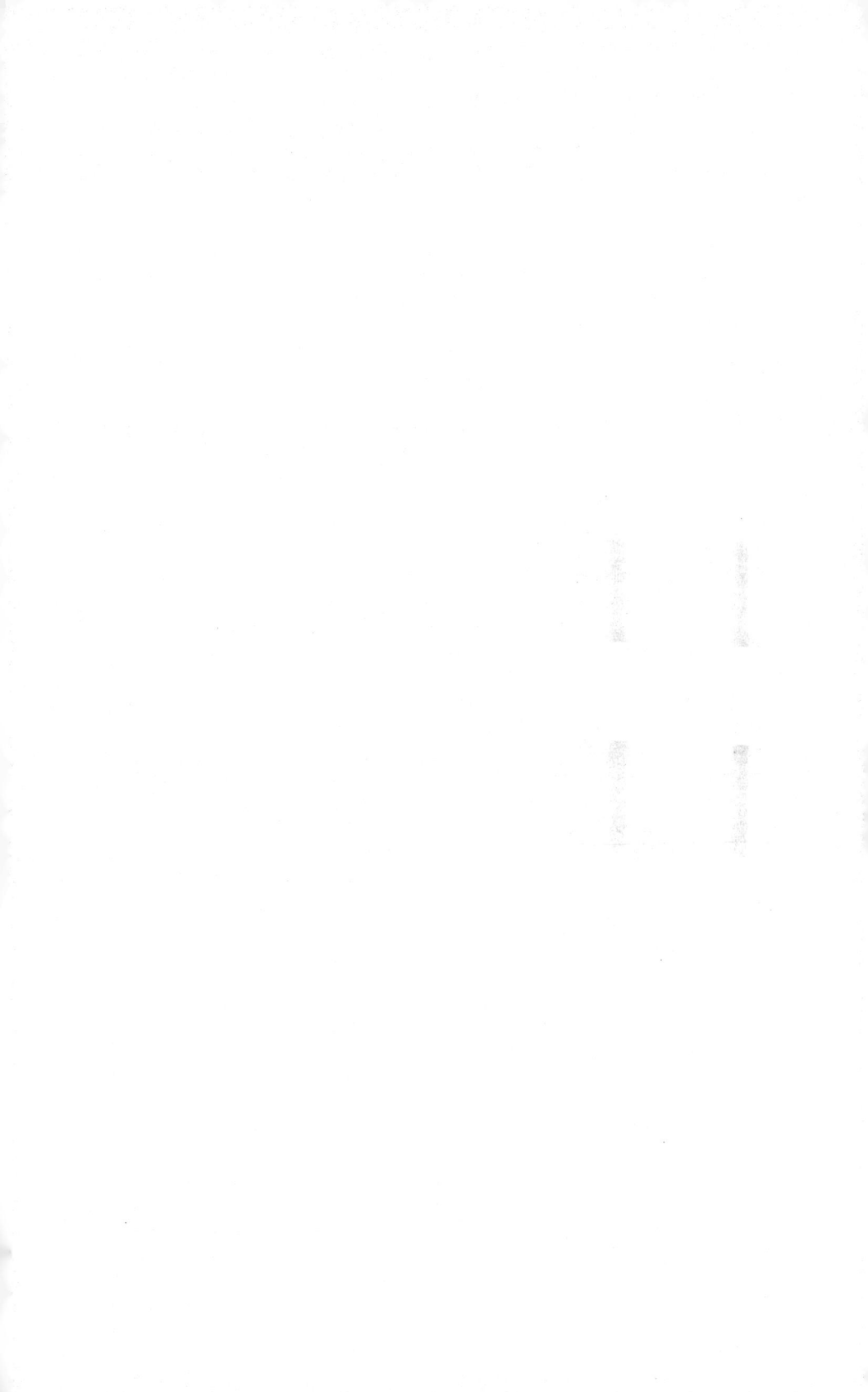

Printed in Great Britain
by Amazon